Biomechanics: An Introduction

Biomechanics: An Introduction

Edited by
Edward Pollock

Larsen & Keller
www.larsen-keller.com

Biomechanics: An Introduction
Edited by Edward Pollock
ISBN: 978-1-63549-725-0 (Hardback)

Larsen & Keller

Published by Larsen and Keller Education,
5 Penn Plaza,
19th Floor,
New York, NY 10001, USA

Cataloging-in-Publication Data

Biomechanics : an introduction / edited by Edward Pollock.
p. cm.
Includes bibliographical references and index.
ISBN 978-1-63549-725-0
1. Biomechanics. 2. Medical sciences. I. Pollock, Edward.
QH513 .B56 2018
571.43--dc23

Printed and bound in China.

For more information regarding Larsen and Keller Education and its products, please visit the publisher's website www.larsen-keller.com

Table of Contents

Preface

The field which uses the laws and rules of mechanics to study the functions of biological systems like plants, animals, humans, fungi, cells, organs, etc. is known as biomechanics. This vast field has many sub-fields like allometry, soft body dynamics, cardiovascular biomechanics, rehabilitation, biofluid mechanics, computational mechanics, kinesiology, animal locomotion, etc. This book unfolds the innovative aspects of biomechanics which will be crucial for the holistic understanding of the subject matter. Some of the diverse topics covered in it address the varied branches that fall under this category. This textbook will serve as a reference to a broad spectrum of readers.

A detailed account of the significant topics covered in this book is provided below:

Chapter 1- The study of the structures of systems found in plants, organs and humans is known as biomechanics. Some of the subfields of biomechanics include kinesiology, animal locomotion and gait analysis, sports biomechanics, biotribology and computational biomechanics. The chapter on biomechanics offers an insightful focus, keeping in mind the complex subject matter.

Chapter 2- The skeleton forms the structure of the body of any organism. They can be of various types like the exoskeleton, endoskeleton, cytoskeleton and hydroskeleton. This chapter provides a plethora of interdisciplinary topics for better comprehension of the biomechanics of the skeleton.

Chapter 3- One of the methods of human locomotion is crawling. The types of crawls are bear crawl, bridge walk, standard crawl, leopard crawl, tiger crawl, etc. Walking and running, trotting, etc. are other forms of human locomotion. This chapter is an overview of the subject matter incorporating all the major aspects of biomechanics.

Chapter 4- Sports biomechanics is the analysis of any form of physical movement displayed in sports in general. Kinematics and kinetics are two important aspects of sports biomechanics. The aspects elucidated in this chapter are of vital importance, and provide a better understanding of biomechanics.

It gives me an immense pleasure to thank our entire team for their efforts. Finally in the end, I would like to thank my family and colleagues who have been a great source of inspiration and support.

Editor

Understanding Biomechanics

The study of the structures of systems found in plants, organs and humans is known as biomechanics. Some of the subfields of biomechanics include kinesiology, animal locomotion and gait analysis, sports biomechanics, biotribology and computational biomechanics. The chapter on biomechanics offers an insightful focus, keeping in mind the complex subject matter.

Biomechanics

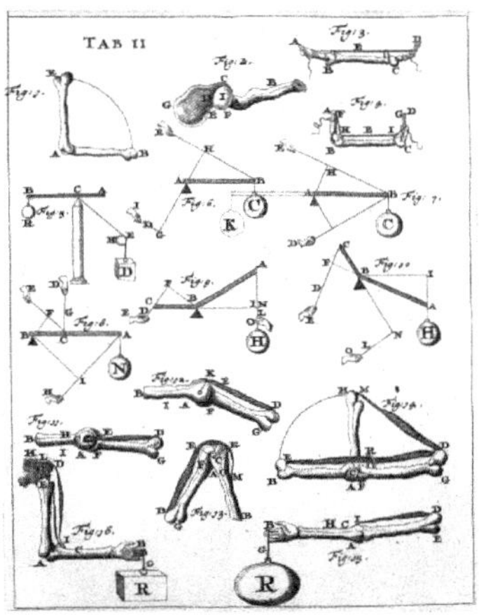

Page of one of the first works of Biomechanics (*De Motu Animalium* of Giovanni Alfonso Borelli) in the 17th century.

Biomechanics is the study of the structure and function of biological systems such as humans, animals, plants, organs, fungi, and cells by means of the methods of mechanics.

Word History

The word "biomechanics" (1899) and the related "biomechanical" (1856) come from the Ancient Greek *bios* "life" and *mēchanikē* "mechanics", to refer to the study of the mechanical principles of living organisms, particularly their movement and structure.

Method

Biomechanics is closely related to engineering, because it often uses traditional engineering sciences to analyze biological systems. Some simple applications of Newtonian mechanics and/or materials sciences can supply correct approximations to the mechanics of many biological systems. Applied mechanics, most notably mechanical engineering disciplines such as continuum mechanics, mechanism analysis, structural analysis, kinematics and dynamics play prominent roles in the study of biomechanics.

Usually biological systems are much more complex than man-built systems. Numerical methods are hence applied in almost every biomechanical study. Research is done in an iterative process of hypothesis and verification, including several steps of modeling, computer simulation and experimental measurements.

Subfields

Applied subfields of biomechanics include:

- Soft body dynamics
- Kinesiology (kinetics + physiology)
- Animal locomotion & Gait analysis
- Musculoskeletal & orthopedic biomechanics
- Cardiovascular biomechanics
- Ergonomy
- Human factors engineering & occupational biomechanics
- Implant (medicine), Orthotics & Prosthesis
- Rehabilitation
- Sports biomechanics
- Allometry
- Injury biomechanics
- Biotribology
- Biofluid mechanics
- Comparative biomechanics
- Computational biomechanics

Sports Biomechanics

In sports biomechanics, the laws of mechanics are applied to human movement in order to gain a greater understanding of athletic performance and to reduce sport injuries as well. It focuses on the application of the scientific principles of mechanical physics to understand movements of action of human bodies and sports implements such as cricket bat, hockey stick and javelin etc. Elements of mechanical engineering (e.g., strain gauges), electrical engineering (e.g., digital filtering), computer science (e.g., numerical methods), gait analysis (e.g., force platforms), and clinical neurophysiology (e.g., surface EMG) are common methods used in sports biomechanics.

Biomechanics in sports can be stated as the muscular, joint and skeletal actions of the body during the execution of a given task, skill and/or technique. Proper understanding of biomechanics relating to sports skill has the greatest implications on: sport's performance, rehabilitation and injury prevention, along with sport mastery. As noted by Doctor Michael Yessis, one could say that best athlete is the one that executes his or her skill the best.

Continuum Biomechanics

The mechanical analysis of biomaterials and biofluids is usually carried forth with the concepts of continuum mechanics. This assumption breaks down when the length scales of interest approach the order of the micro structural details of the material. One of the most remarkable characteristic of biomaterials is their hierarchical structure. In other words, the mechanical characteristics of these materials rely on physical phenomena occurring in multiple levels, from the molecular all the way up to the tissue and organ levels.

Biomaterials are classified in two groups, hard and soft tissues. Mechanical deformation of hard tissues (like wood, shell and bone) may be analysed with the theory of linear elasticity. On the other hand, soft tissues (like skin, tendon, muscle and cartilage) usually undergo large deformations and thus their analysis rely on the finite strain theory and computer simulations. The interest in continuum biomechanics is spurred by the need for realism in the development of medical simulation.

Biofluid Mechanics

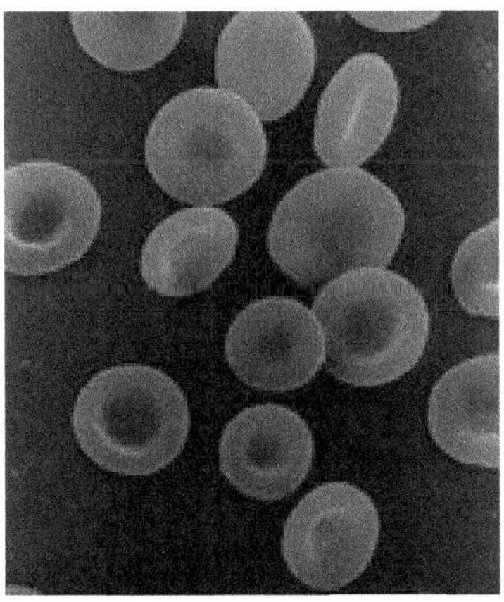

Red blood cells

Biological fluid mechanics, or biofluid mechanics, is the study of both gas and liquid fluid flows in or around biological organisms. An often studied liquid biofluids problem is that of blood flow in the human cardiovascular system. Under certain mathematical circumstances, blood flow can be modelled by the Navier–Stokes equations. *In vivo* whole blood is assumed to be an incompressible Newtonian fluid. However, this assumption fails when considering forward flow within arterioles. At the microscopic scale, the effects of individual red blood cells become significant, and whole blood can no longer be modelled as a continuum. When the diameter of the blood vessel is just slightly larger than the diameter of the red blood cell the Fahraeus–Lindquist effect occurs and there is a decrease in wall shear stress. However, as the diameter of the blood vessel decreases further, the red blood cells have to squeeze through the vessel and often can only pass in single file. In this case, the inverse Fahraeus–Lindquist effect occurs and the wall shear stress increases.

An example of a gaseous biofluids problem is that of human respiration. Recently, respiratory systems in insects have been studied for bioinspiration for designing improved microfluidic devices.

Biotribology

The main aspects of Contact mechanics and tribology are related to friction, wear and lubrication. When the two surfaces come in contact during motion i.e. rub against each other, friction, wear and lubrication effects are very important to analyze in order to determine the performance of the material. Biotribology is a study of friction, wear and lubrication of biological systems especially human joints such as hips and knees. For example, femoral and tibial components of knee implant routinely rub against each other during daily activity such as walking or stair climbing. If the performance of tibial component needs to be analyzed, the principles of biotribology are used to determine the wear performance of the implant and lubrication effects of synovial fluid. In addition, the theory of contact mechanics also becomes very important for wear analysis. Additional aspects of biotribology can also include analysis of subsurface damage resulting from two surfaces coming in contact during motion, i.e. rubbing against each other, such as in the evaluation of tissue engineered cartilage.

Comparative Biomechanics

Comparative biomechanics is the application of biomechanics to non-human organisms, whether used to gain greater insights into humans (as in physical anthropology) or into the functions, ecology and adaptations of the organisms themselves. Common areas of investigation are Animal locomotion and feeding, as these have strong connections to the organism's fitness and impose high mechanical demands. Animal locomotion, has many manifestations, including running, jumping and flying. Locomotion requires energy to overcome friction, drag, inertia, and gravity, though which factor predominates varies with environment.

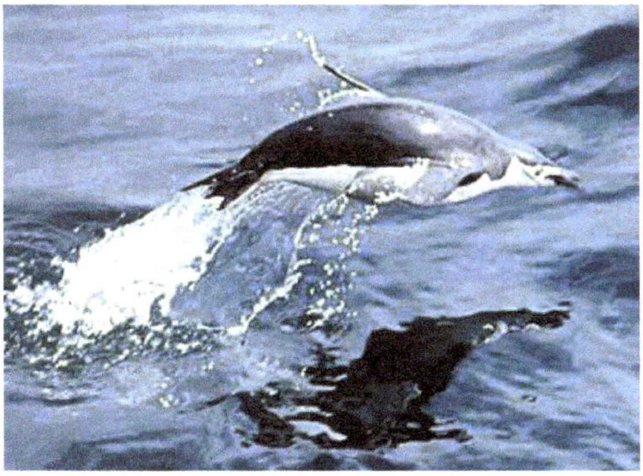

Chinstrap penguin leaping over water

Comparative biomechanics overlaps strongly with many other fields, including ecology, neurobiology, developmental biology, ethology, and paleontology, to the extent of commonly publishing papers in the journals of these other fields. Comparative biomechanics is often applied in medicine (with regards to common model organisms such as mice and rats) as well as in biomimetics, which looks to nature for solutions to engineering problems.

Plant Biomechanics

The application of biomechanical principles to plants and plant organs has developed into the subfield of plant biomechanics.

Computational Biomechanics

Over the past decade the Finite element method has become an established alternative to in vivo surgical assessment. The main advantage of Computational Biomechanics lies in its ability to determine the endo-anatomical response of an anatomy, without being subject to ethical restrictions. This has led FE modelling to the point of becoming ubiquitous in several fields of Biomechanics while several projects have even adopted an open source philosophy (e.g. BioSpine).

History

Antiquity

Aristotle wrote the first book on the motion of animals, *De Motu Animalium*, or On the Movement of Animals. He not only saw animals' bodies as mechanical systems, but pursued questions such as the physiological difference between imagining performing an action and actually doing it. In another work, *On the Parts of Animals*, he provided an accurate description of how the ureter uses peristalsis to carry urine from the kidneys to the bladder.

Renaissance

Leonardo da Vinci studied anatomy in the context of mechanics. He analyzed muscle forces as acting along lines connecting origins and insertions, and studied joint function. Da Vinci tended to mimic some animal features in his machines. For example, he studied the flight of birds to find means by which humans could fly; and because horses were the principal source of mechanical power in that time, he studied their muscular systems to design machines that would better benefit from the forces applied by this animal.

Galileo Galilei was interested in the strength of bones and suggested that bones are hollow because this affords maximum strength with minimum weight. He noted that animals' bone masses increased disproportionately to their size. Consequently, bones must also increase disproportionately in girth rather than mere size. This is because the bending strength of a tubular structure (such as a bone) is much more efficient relative to its weight. Mason suggests that this insight was one of the first grasps of the principles of biological optimization.

In the 16th century, Descartes suggested a philosophic system whereby all living systems, including the human body (but not the soul), are simply machines ruled by the same mechanical laws, an idea that did much to promote and sustain biomechanical study. Giovanni Alfonso Borelli embraced this idea and studied walking, running, jumping, the flight of birds, the swimming of fish, and even the piston action of the heart within a mechanical framework. He could determine the position of the human center of gravity, calculate and measured inspired and expired air volumes, and showed that inspiration is muscle-driven and expiration is due to tissue elasticity. Borelli was the first to understand that the levers of the musculoskeletal system magnify motion rather than force, so that muscles must produce much larger forces than those resisting the motion. Influenced by the work of Galileo, whom he personally knew, he had an intuitive understanding of static equilibrium in various joints of the human body well before Newton published the laws of motion.

Industrial Era

In the 19th century Étienne-Jules Marey used cinematography to scientifically investigate locomotion. He opened the field of modern 'motion analysis' by being the first to correlate ground reaction forces with movement. In Germany, the brothers Ernst Heinrich Weber and Wilhelm Eduard Weber hypothesized a great deal about human gait, but it was Christian Wilhelm Braune who significantly advanced the science using recent advances in engineering mechanics. During the same period, the engineering mechanics of materials began to flourish in France and Germany under the demands of the industrial revolution. This led to the rebirth of bone biomechanics when the railroad engineer Karl Culmann and the anatomist Hermann von Meyer compared the stress patterns in a human femur with those in a similarly shaped crane. Inspired by this finding Julius Wolff proposed the famous Wolff's law of bone remodeling.

Applications

The study of biomechanics ranges from the inner workings of a cell to the movement and development of limbs, to the mechanical properties of soft tissue, and bones. Some simple examples of biomechanics research include the investigation of the forces that act on limbs, the aerodynamics of bird and insect flight, the hydrodynamics of swimming in fish, and locomotion in general across all forms of life, from individual cells to whole organisms. The biomechanics of human beings is a core part of kinesiology. As we develop a greater understanding of the physiological behavior of living tissues, researchers are able to advance the field of tissue engineering, as well as develop improved treatments for a wide array of pathologies.

Biomechanics is also applied to studying human musculoskeletal systems. Such research utilizes force platforms to study human ground reaction forces and infrared videography to capture the trajectories of markers attached to the human body to study human 3D motion. Research also applies electromyography (EMG) system to study the muscle activation. By this, it is feasible to investigate the muscle responses to the external forces as well as perturbations.

Biomechanics is widely used in orthopedic industry to design orthopedic implants for human joints, dental parts, external fixations and other medical purposes. Biotribology is a very important part of it. It is a study of the performance and function of biomaterials used for orthopedic implants. It plays a vital role to improve the design and produce successful biomaterials for medical and clinical purposes. One such example is in tissue engineered cartilage.

References

- Christian, A.; Garland T., Jr. (1996). "Scaling of limb proportions in monitor lizards (Squamata: Varanidae)" (PDF). Journal of Herpetology. 30 (2): 219–230. JSTOR 1565513. doi:10.2307/1565513
- Longo, Giuseppe; Montévil, Maël (2014-01-01). Perspectives on Organisms. Lecture Notes in Morphogenesis. Springer Berlin Heidelberg. pp. 23–73. ISBN 9783642359378. doi:10.1007/978-3-642-35938-5_2
- Otto Snell (1892). "Die Abhängigkeit des Hirngewichts von dem Körpergewicht und den geistigen Fähigkeiten". Arch. Psychiatr. 23 (2): 436–446. doi:10.1007/BF01843462
- Kerkhoff, A.J.; Enquist, B.J. (2009). "Multiplicative by nature: Why logarithmic transformation is necessary in allometry". Journal of Theoretical Biology. 257 (3): 519–521. doi:10.1016/j.jtbi.2008.12.026
- Vogel, Steven (1988). Life's Devices : The Physical World of Animals and Plants. Princeton University Press. p. 39. ISBN 978-0-691-02418-9. Retrieved 29 March 2014
- O'Hara, R.B.; Kotze, D.J. (2010). "Do not log-transform count data". Methods in Ecology and Evolution. 1 (2): 118–122. doi:10.1111/j.2041-210X.2010.00021.x

- Garland Jr., T. (1983). "The relation between maximal running speed and body mass in terrestrial mammals" (PDF). Journal of Zoology, London. 199 (2): 157–170. doi:10.1111/j.1469-7998.1983.tb02087.x
- Schmidt-Nielsen, Knut (10 April 1997). Animal Physiology: Adaptation and Environment (5th ed.). Cambridge University Press. ISBN 978-0-521-57098-5
- Roberts, Thomas J.; Azizi, Emanuel (2011). "Flexible mechanisms: the diverse roles of biological springs in vertebrate movement". The Journal of Experimental Biology. 214 (3): 353–361. PMC 3020146. PMID 21228194. doi:10.1242/jeb.038588
- Bornstein MH, Bornstein HG (19 February 1976). "The Pace of Life". Nature. 259 (5544): 557–9. Bibcode:1976Natur.259..557B. doi:10.1038/259557a0

2

Biomechanics of the Skeleton

The skeleton forms the structure of the body of any organism. They can be of various types like the exoskeleton, endoskeleton, cytoskeleton and hydroskeleton. This chapter provides a plethora of interdisciplinary topics for better comprehension of the biomechanics of the skeleton.

Skeleton

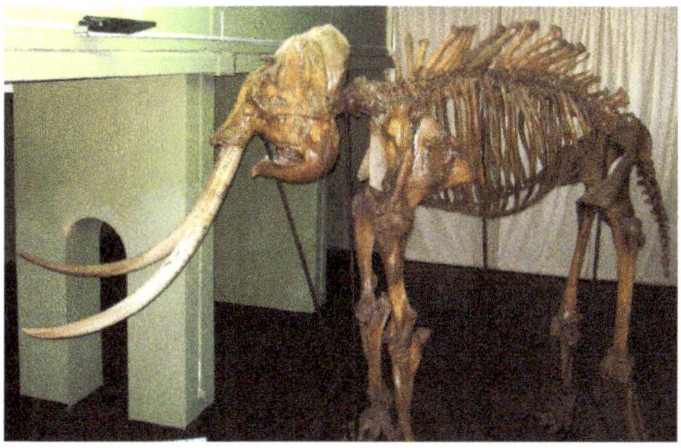

Heiyantuduwa Raja (elephant) Skeleton at National Museum of Colombo Sri Lanka.

The skeleton is the body part that forms the supporting structure of an organism. There are several different skeletal types: the exoskeleton, which is the stable outer shell of an organism, the endoskeleton, which forms the support structure inside the body, the hydroskeleton, and the cytoskeleton.

Types of Skeletons

There are two major types of skeletons: solid and fluid. Solid skeletons can be internal, called an endoskeleton, or external, called an exoskeleton, and may be further classified as pliant (elastic/movable) or rigid (hard/non-movable). Fluid skeletons are always internal.

Exoskeleton

Exoskeletons are external, and are found in many invertebrates; they enclose and protect the soft tissues and organs of the body. Some kinds of exoskeletons undergo periodic moulting as the animal grows, as is the case in many arthropods including insects and crustaceans.

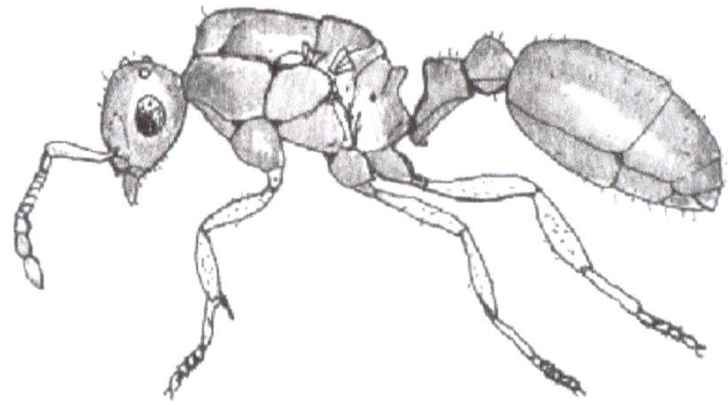

Exoskeleton of an ant

The exoskeleton of insects is not only a form of protection, but also serves as a surface for muscle attachment, as a watertight protection against drying, and as a sense organ to interact with the environment. The shell of mollusks also performs all of the same functions, except that in most cases it does not contain sense organs.

An external skeleton can be quite heavy in relation to the overall mass of an animal, so on land, organisms that have an exoskeleton are mostly relatively small. Somewhat larger aquatic animals can support an exoskeleton because weight is less of a consideration underwater. The southern giant clam, a species of extremely large saltwater clam in the Pacific Ocean, has a shell that is massive in both size and weight. *Syrinx aruanus* is a species of sea snail with a very large shell.

Endoskeleton

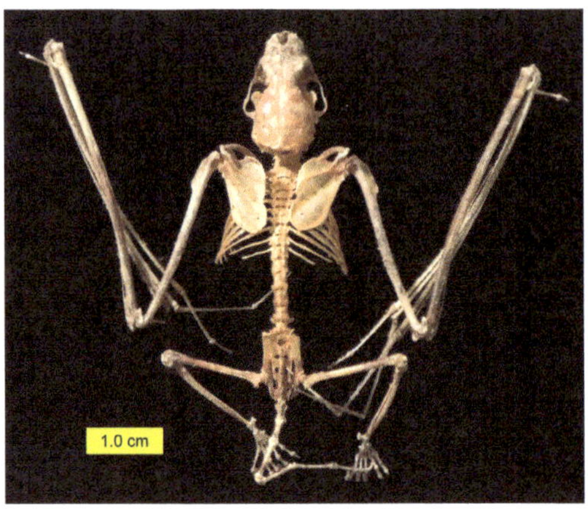

Endoskeleton of a bat

The endoskeleton is the internal support structure of an animal, composed of mineralized tissue and is typical of vertebrates. Endoskeletons vary in complexity from functioning purely for support (as in the case of sponges), to serving as an attachment site for muscles and a mechanism for transmitting muscular forces. A true endoskeleton is derived from mesodermal tissue. Such a skeleton is present in echinoderms and chordates.

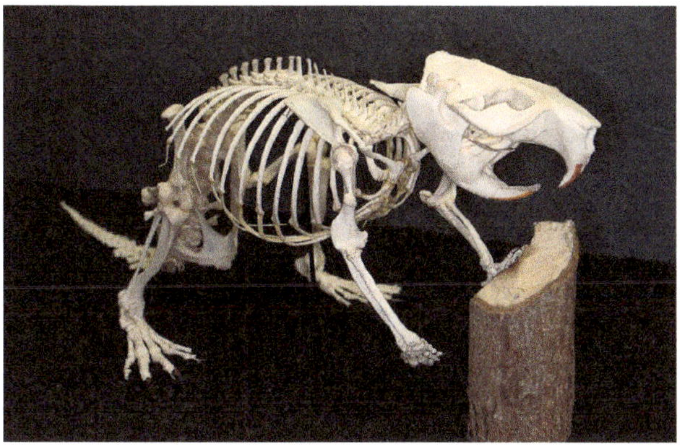

A beaver skeleton on display at The Museum of Osteology, Oklahoma City, Oklahoma.

Pliant Skeletons

Pliant skeletons are capable of movement; thus, when stress is applied to the skeletal structure, it deforms and then reverts to its original shape. This skeletal structure is used in some invertebrates, for instance in the hinge of bivalve shells or the mesoglea of cnidarians such as jellyfish. Pliant skeletons are beneficial because only muscle contractions are needed to bend the skeleton; upon muscle relaxation, the skeleton will return to its original shape. Cartilage is one material that a pliant skeleton may be composed of, but most pliant skeletons are formed from a mixture of proteins, polysaccharides, and water. For additional structure or protection, pliant skeletons may be supported by rigid skeletons. Organisms that have pliant skeletons typically live in water, which supports body structure in the absence of a rigid skeleton.

Rigid Skeletons

Rigid skeletons are not capable of movement when stressed, creating a strong support system most common in terrestrial animals. Such a skeleton type used by animals that live in water are more for protection (such as barnacle and snail shells) or for fast-moving animals that require additional support of musculature needed for swimming through water. Rigid skeletons are formed from materials including chitin (in arthropods), calcium compounds such as calcium carbonate (in stony corals and mollusks) and silicate (for diatoms and radiolarians).

Cytoskeleton

The cytoskeleton (gr. *kytos* = cell) is used to stabilize and preserve the form of the cells. It is a dynamic structure that maintains cell shape, protects the cell, enables cellular motion (using structures such as flagella, cilia and lamellipodia), and plays important roles in both intracellular transport (the movement of vesicles and organelles, for example) and cellular division.

Fluid Skeletons

A hydrostatic skeleton is a semi-rigid, soft tissue structure filled with liquid under pressure, surrounded by muscles. Longitudinal and circular muscles around their body sectors allow movement by alternate lengthening and contractions along their lengths. A common example of this is earthworm.

Organisms with Skeletons

Invertebrates

The endoskeletons of echinoderms and some other soft-bodied invertebrates such as jellyfish and earthworms are also termed hydrostatic; a body cavity the coelom is filled with coelomic fluid and the pressure from this fluid acts together with the surrounding muscles to change the organism's shape and produce movement.

Sponges

The skeleton of sponges consists of microscopic calcareous or silicious spicules. The demosponges include 90% of all species of sponges. Their "skeletons" are made of spicules consisting of fibers of the protein spongin, the mineral silica, or both. Where spicules of silica are present, they have a different shape from those in the otherwise similar glass sponges.

Echinoderms

The skeleton of the echinoderms, which include, among other things, the starfish, is composed of calcite and a small amount of magnesium oxide. It lies below the epidermis in the mesoderm and is within cell clusters of frame-forming cells. This structure formed is porous and therefore firm and at the same time light. It coalesces into small calcareous ossicles (bony plates), which can grow in all directions and thus can replace the loss of a body part. Connected by joints, the individual skeletal parts can be moved by the muscles.

Vertebrates

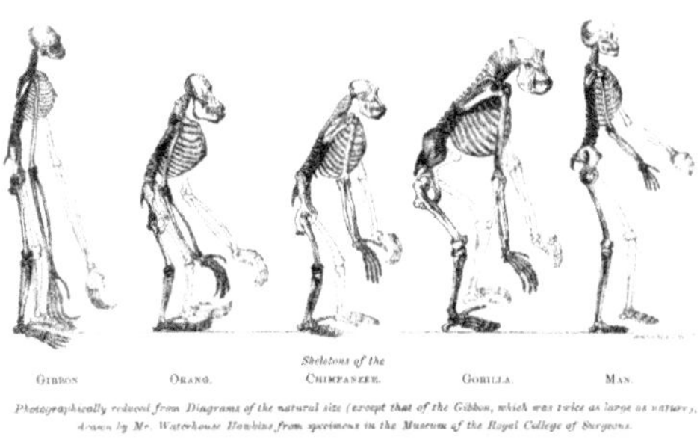

Pithecometra: From Thomas Huxley's 1863 *Evidence as to Man's Place in Nature*, the compared skeletons of apes to humans.

In most vertebrates, the main skeletal component is referred to as bone. Another important component is cartilage which in mammals is found mainly in the joint areas. In other animals, such as the cartilaginous fishes, which include the sharks, the skeleton is composed entirely of cartilage. The segmental pattern of the skeleton is present in all vertebrates (mammals, birds, fish, reptiles and amphibians) with basic units being repeated. This segmental pattern is particularly evident in the vertebral column and the ribcage.

Bones in addition to supporting the body also serve, at the cellular level, as calcium and phosphate storage.

Fish

The skeleton, which forms the support structure inside the fish is either made of cartilage as in the (Chondrichthyes), or bones as in the (Osteichthyes). The main skeletal element is the vertebral column, composed of articulating vertebrae which are lightweight yet strong. The ribs attach to the spine and there are no limbs or limb girdles. They are supported only by the muscles. The main external features of the fish, the fins, are composed of either bony or soft spines called rays, which with the exception of the caudal fin (tail fin), have no direct connection with the spine. They are supported by the muscles which compose the main part of the trunk.

Birds

The bird skeleton is highly adapted for flight. It is extremely lightweight, yet still strong enough to withstand the stresses of taking off, flying, and landing. One key adaptation is the fusing of bones into single ossifications, such as the pygostyle. Because of this, birds usually have a smaller number of bones than other terrestrial vertebrates. Birds also lack teeth or even a true jaw, instead having evolved a beak, which is far more lightweight. The beaks of many baby birds have a projection called an egg tooth, which facilitates their exit from the amniotic egg.

Marine Mammals

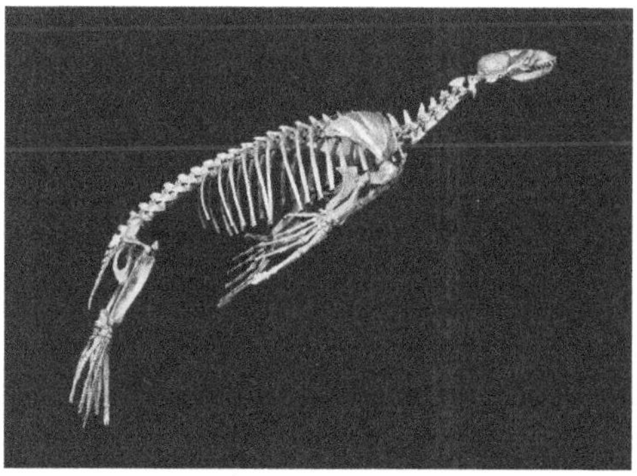

Californian sea lion

To facilitate the movement of marine mammals in water, the hind legs were either lost altogether, as in the whales and manatees, or united in a single tail fin as in the pinnipeds (seals). In the whale, the cervical vertebrae are typically fused, an adaptation trading flexibility for stability during swimming.

Humans

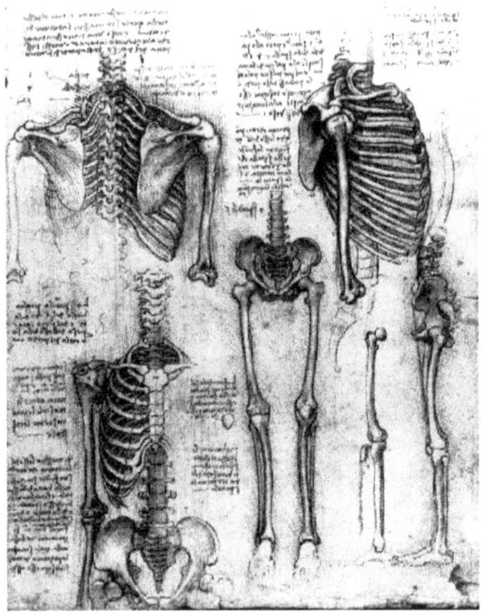

Study of Skeletons, c. 1510, by Leonardo da Vinci.

The human skeleton consists of both fused and individual bones supported and supplemented by ligaments, tendons, muscles and cartilage. It serves as a scaffold which supports organs, anchors muscles, and protects organs such as the brain, lungs, heart and spinal cord. Although the teeth do not consist of tissue commonly found in bones, the teeth are usually considered as members of the skeletal system. The biggest bone in the body is the femur in the upper leg, and the smallest is the stapes bone in the middle ear. In an adult, the skeleton comprises around 14% of the total body weight, and half of this weight is water.

Fused bones include those of the pelvis and the cranium. Not all bones are interconnected directly: There are three bones in each middle ear called the ossicles that articulate only with each other. The hyoid bone, which is located in the neck and serves as the point of attachment for the tongue, does not articulate with any other bones in the body, being supported by muscles and ligaments.

There are 206 bones in the adult human skeleton, although this number depends on whether the pelvic bones (the hip bones on each side) are counted as one or three bones on each side (ilium, ischium, and pubis), whether the coccyx or tail bone is counted as one or four separate bones, and does not count the variable wormian bones between skull sutures. Similarly, the sacrum is usually counted as a single bone, rather than five fused vertebrae. There is also a variable number of small sesamoid bones, commonly found in tendons. The patella or kneecap on each side is an example of a larger sesamoid bone. The patellae are counted in the total, as they are constant. The number of bones varies between individuals and with age - newborn babies have over 270 bones some of which fuse together. These bones are organized into a longitudinal axis, the axial skeleton, to which the appendicular skeleton is attached.

The human skeleton takes 20 years before it is fully developed. In many animals, the skeleton bones contain marrow, which produces blood cells.

There exist several general differences between the male and female skeletons. The male skeleton, for example, is generally larger and heavier than the female skeleton. In the female skeleton, the bones of the skull are generally less angular. The female skeleton also has wider and shorter breastbone and slimmer wrists. There exist significant differences between the male and female pelvis which are related to the female's pregnancy and childbirth capabilities. The female pelvis is wider and shallower than the male pelvis. Female pelvises also have an enlarged pelvic outlet and a wider and more circular pelvic inlet. The angle between the pubic bones is known to be sharper in males, which results in a more circular, narrower, and near heart-shaped pelvis.

Bones and Cartilage

Bone

Bones are rigid organs that form part of the endoskeleton of vertebrates. They function to move, support, and protect the various organs of the body, produce red and white blood cells and store minerals. Bone tissue is a type of dense connective tissue. Bones have a variety of shapes with a complex internal and external structure they are also lightweight, yet strong and hard. One of the types of tissue that makes up bone tissue is mineralized tissue and this gives it rigidity and a honeycomb-like three-dimensional internal structure. Other types of tissue found in bones include marrow, endosteum and periosteum, nerves, blood vessels and cartilage. There are 206 bones in the adult human body and 270 in an infant.

Cartilage

During embryogenesis the precursor to bone development is cartilage. Much of this substance is then replaced by bone during the second and third trimester, after the flesh such as muscle has formed around it; forming the skeleton. Cartilage is a stiff and inflexible connective tissue found in many areas in the bodies of humans and other animals, including the joints between bones, the rib cage, the ear, the nose, the elbow, the knee, the ankle, the bronchial tubes and the intervertebral discs. It is not as hard and rigid as bone but is stiffer and less flexible than muscle.

Cartilage is composed of specialized cells called chondrocytes that produce a large amount of extracellular matrix composed of Type II collagen (except Fibrocartilage which also contains type I collagen) fibers, abundant ground substance rich in proteoglycan, and elastin fibers. Cartilage is classified in three types, elastic cartilage, hyaline cartilage and fibrocartilage, which differ in the relative amounts of these three main components.

Unlike other connective tissues, cartilage does not contain blood vessels. The chondrocytes are supplied by diffusion, helped by the pumping action generated by compression of the articular cartilage or flexion of the elastic cartilage. Thus, compared to other connective tissues, cartilage grows and repairs more slowly.

In Popular Culture

In Western culture, the skeleton is oftentimes seen as a fearful symbol of death and the paranormal. It is a popular motif in the holiday Halloween, as well as Day of the Dead.

Hydrostatic Skeleton

A hydrostatic skeleton, or hydroskeleton, is a skeleton supported by fluid pressure. Hydrostatic skeletons are common among simple invertebrate organisms. While more advanced organisms can be considered hydrostatic, they are sometimes referred to as hydrostatic for their possession of a hydrostatic organ instead of a hydrostatic skeleton. A hydrostatic organ and a hydrostatic skeleton may have the same capabilities, but they are not the same. Hydrostatic organs are more common in advanced organisms, while hydrostatic skeletons are more common in primitive organisms. As its name suggests, containing hydro meaning "water", being hydrostatic means that the skeleton or organ is fluid-filled.

As a skeletal structure, it possesses the ability to affect shape and movement, and involves two mechanical units: the muscle layers and the body wall. The muscular layers are longitudinal and circular, and part of the fluid- filled coelom within. Contractions of the circular muscles lengthen the organism's body, while contractions of the longitudinal muscles shorten the organism's body. Fluid within the organism is evenly concentrated so the forces of the muscle are spread throughout the whole organism and shape changes can persist. These structural factors also persist in a hydrostatic organ.

University of Massachusetts researcher Diane Kelly documents a non-helical hydrostatic skeleton structure as the functional basis of the mammalian penis which must function similarly to a rigid element in use. Helically reinforced hydrostatic skeleton structure is typical for flexible structures as in soft-bodied animals.

Structure

Hydrostatic skeletons are typically arranged in a cylinder. Hydrostatic skeletons can be controlled by several different muscle types. Length can be adjusted by longitudinal muscle fibers parallel to the longitudinal axis. The muscle fibers may be found in continuous sheets or isolated bundles, and the diameter can be manipulated by three different muscle types: circular, radial, and transverse. Circular musculature wraps around the circumference of the cylinder, radial musculature extends from the center of the cylinder towards the surface, and transverse musculature arrange in parallel and perpendicular sheets crossing the diameter of the cylinder.

Within the cylinder lies fluid, most often water. The fluid resists to changes in volume. Contraction of circular, radial or transverse muscles increases the pressure within the cylinder, and results in an increase in length. Contraction of longitudinal muscles can shorten the cylinder.

Change in shape is limited by connective tissue fibers. Connective fibers, often collagenous, are arranged in a helical shape within the wall of the hydrostatic skeleton. The helical shape formed by these fibers allows for elongation and shortening of the skeleton, while still remaining rigid to prevent torsion. As the shape of the cylinder changes, the pitch of the helix will change. The angle relative to the long axis will decrease during elongation and increase during shortening.

Advantages and Disadvantages

Organisms containing a hydrostatic skeleton have advantages and disadvantages. Their fluid shape allows them to move around easily while swimming and burrowing. They can fit through oddly shaped passages and hide themselves more effectively from predators. They are able to create a force when squeezing through rocks and create a "prying open" gesture. There is a lightweight, flexible component to them that allows this movement with very little muscle mass.

These organisms are also able to heal faster than organisms that contain hard skeletons. Healing in these organisms varies from creature to creature. However, if the cavity needs to be refilled, the "fluid" can easily be refilled if it is water or blood. If the fluid is some other type of liquid, it can take longer, but it is still faster than healing a bone. The common earthworm is also able to regrow damaged parts of their body.

These organisms have some relatively simple pathways for circulation and respiration. Also, these organisms have a cushion to allow protection for internal organs from shock. However, it does not protect internal organs from external damage very effectively.

Because the hydrostatic skeletons have limited ability for attachment of limbs, the organisms are relatively simple and do not have many abilities to grab or latch onto things. Organisms with complete hydrostatic skeletons need to be in an environment that allows them to re-fill themselves with their fluid that is necessary for survival. This is why hydrostatic skeletons are common in marine life. They have a large amount of access to the necessary elements for survival. Terrestrial organisms that have hydrostatic skeletons generally have a lack of strength because they are not in a fluid environment. If they were to expand their body too much, they would collapse under their own weight.

Organisms

Hydrostatic skeletons are very common in invertebrates. A common example is the earthworm. Also, hydrostatic nature is common in marine life such as jelly fish, starfish, and sea anemones. Earthworms have rings of muscles that are filled with fluid, making their entire body hydrostatic. A sea anemone has a hydrostatic head, with arms radiating out around the mouth. This structure is helpful in feeding and locomotion.

An example of a simple vertebrate containing a hydrostatic skeleton would be Enteropneusta, with the common name of acorn worm. This organism is classified as a Hemichordate, and they are marine worms that use their hydrostatic skeleton to tunnel and anchor themselves into the ground. This can be used for locomotion, but also can aid in the defense of the organism against outside forces as the worm can try to "hide" itself within the ocean floor.

Vertebrates

The function of the mammalian penis relies on the use of a hydrostatic skeleton and is known as a hydrostatic organ. The hydrostatic fluid, which in this case is blood, fills the penis during an erection. Unlike the use of hydrostatic skeletons in many invertebrates, which use the bending of the animal for locomotion, the penis must resist bending and shape changes during sexual intercourse. Instead of connective fibers arranged in a helical shape, the penis contains a layer called the corpus cavernosum. The corpus cavernosum contains connective fibers arranged both parallel and perpendicular to the longitudinal axis. These fibers remain folded when the penis is flaccid, but unfold as the penis fills with blood during an erection, which allows the penis to resist bending. The penises of turtles are structured similarly, although they evolved separately.

Other vertebrates sometimes utilize a modified hydrostatic skeleton called a muscular hydrostat. Muscular hydrostats do not contain a fluid-filled cavity. These structures are constructed of muscle and connective fibers, densely packed into a 3-D structure. In many cases, the muscular hydrostat can be manipulated in all three dimensions. This allows for more precise movement compared to a typical hydrostatic skeleton. While in typical hydrostatic skeletons, movement is generated by applying force to a fluid-filled cavity, muscular hydrostats generate movement by muscle contractions. When one muscle contracts and decreases in area, other muscles within the structure must expand in response. Helical muscles may be present, which can create torsion, an ability that is restricted in hydrostatic skeletons. Muscular hydrostats are found in mammalian, reptilian, and amphibian tongues. Mammalian tongues have the structure of a central core of muscle fibers surrounded by bundles of longitudinal muscles and alternating parallel sheets of transverse muscle fibers. Elephant trunks and tapir proboscises also utilize a muscular hydrostat. These structures are composed of longitudinal fibers surrounded by radial and helical fibers.

Cytoskeleton

A cytoskeleton is present in all cells of all domains of life (archaea, bacteria, eukaryotes). It is a complex network of interlinking filaments and tubules that extend throughout the cytoplasm, from the nucleus to the plasma membrane. The cytoskeletal systems of different organisms are composed of similar proteins. In eukaryotes, the cytoskeletal matrix is a dynamic structure composed of three main proteins, which are capable of rapid growth or disassembly dependent on the cell's requirements at a certain period of time.

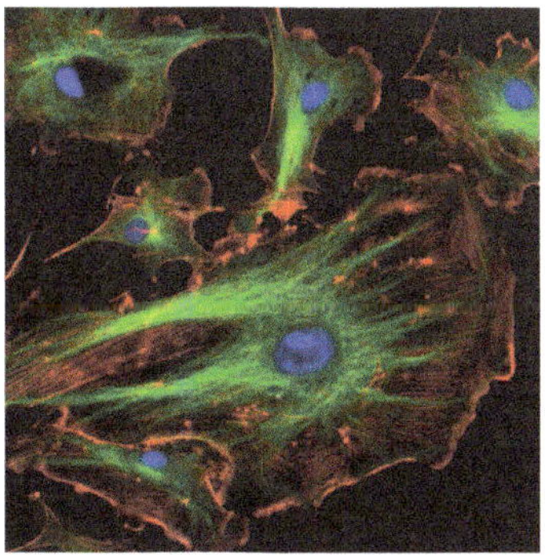

The eukaryotic cytoskeleton. Actin filaments are shown in red, and microtubules composed of beta tubulin are in green.

The structure, function and dynamic behaviour of the cytoskeleton can be very different, depending on organism and cell type. Even within one cell the cytoskeleton can change through association with other proteins and the previous history of the network.

There is a multitude of functions that the cytoskeleton can perform. Primarily, it gives the cell its shape and mechanical resistance to deformation, and through association with extracellular connective tissue and other cells it stabilizes entire tissues. The cytoskeleton can also contract, thereby deforming the cell and the cell's environment and allowing cells to migrate. Moreover, it is involved in many cell signaling pathways, in the uptake of extracellular material (endocytosis), segregates chromosomes during cellular division, is involved in cytokinesis (the division of a mother cell into two daughter cells), provides a scaffold to organize the contents of the cell in space and for intracellular transport (for example, the movement of vesicles and organelles within the cell); and can be a template for the construction of a cell wall. Furthermore, it forms specialized structures, such as flagella, cilia, lamellipodia and podosomes.

A large-scale example of an action performed by the cytoskeleton is muscle contraction. During contraction of a muscle, within each muscle cell, myosin molecular motors collectively exert forces on parallel actin filaments. This action contracts the muscle cell, and through the synchronous process in many muscle cells, the entire muscle.

History

In 1903, Nikolai K. Koltsov proposed that the shape of cells was determined by a network of tubules that he termed the cytoskeleton. The concept of a protein mosaic that dynamically coordinated cytoplasmic biochemistry was proposed by Rudolph Peters in 1929 while the term (*cytosquelette*, in French) was first introduced by French embryologist Paul Wintrebert in 1931.

Eukaryotic Cytoskeleton

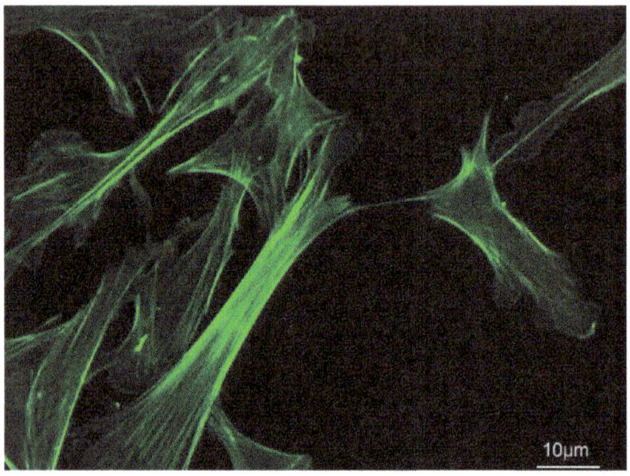

Actin cytoskeleton of mouse embryo fibroblasts, stained with phalloidin.

Eukaryotic cells contain three main kinds of cytoskeletal filaments: microfilaments, microtubules, and intermediate filaments. Each cytoskeletal filament type is formed by polymerization of a distinct type of protein subunit and has its own characteristic shape and intracellular distribution. Microfilaments are polymers of the protein actin and are 7 nm in diameter. Microtubules are composed of tubulin and are 25 nm in diameter. Intermediate filaments are composed of various proteins, depending on the type of cell in which they are found; they are normally 8-12 nm in diameter. The cytoskeleton provides the cell with structure and shape, and by excluding macromolecules from some of the cytosol, it adds to the level of macromolecular crowding in this compartment. Cytoskeletal elements interact extensively and intimately with cellular membranes. A number of small-molecule cytoskeletal drugs have been discovered that interact with actin and microtubules. These compounds have proven useful in studying the cytoskeleton and several have clinical applications. Recently, disassembly-promoting, encodable actin tools (DeActs), genetically encoded actin-modifying polypeptides, which induce actin disassembly in eukaryotic cells, were developed.

All filaments interact with accessory proteins that regulate and link the filaments to other cell compounds and each other. The accessory proteins are essential for controlled assembly of cytoskeletal filaments in particular locations, and they include motor proteins.

Microfilaments (Actin Filaments)

Microfilaments are composed of linear polymers of G-actin proteins, and generate force when the growing (plus) end of the filament pushes against a barrier, such as the cell membrane. They also act as tracks for the movement of myosin molecules that attach to the microfilament and "walk" along them. Myosin motoring along F-actin filaments generates contractile forces in so-called actomyosin fibers, both in muscle as well as most non-muscle cell types. Actin structures are controlled by the Rho family of small GTP-binding proteins such as Rho itself for contractile acto-myosin filaments ("stress fibers"), Rac for lamellipodia and Cdc42 for filopodia.

Intermediate Filaments

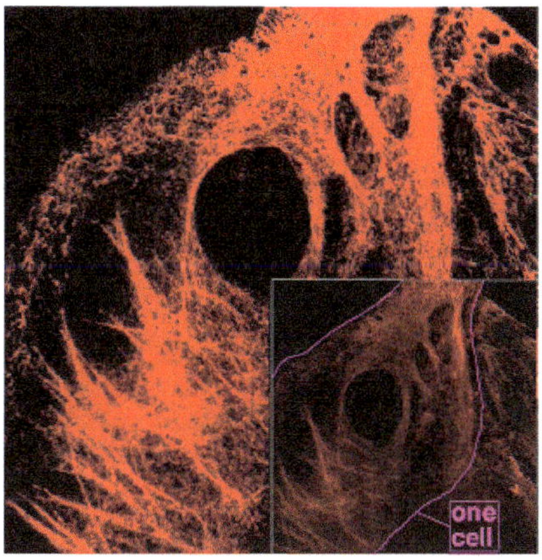

Microscopy of keratin filaments inside cells

Intermediate filaments are a part of the cytoskeleton of all animals. These filaments, averaging 10 nanometers in diameter, are more stable (strongly bound) than actin filaments, and heterogeneous constituents of the cytoskeleton. Like actin filaments, they function in the maintenance of cell-shape by bearing tension (microtubules, by contrast, resist compression but can also bear tension during mitosis and during the positioning of the centrosome). Intermediate filaments organize the internal tridimensional structure of the cell, anchoring organelles and serving as structural components of the nuclear lamina. They also participate in some cell-cell and cell-matrix junctions. Nuclear lamina exist in all animals and all tissues. Some animals like the fruit fly do not have any cytoplasmic intermediate filaments. In those animals that express cytoplasmic intermediate filaments, these are tissue specific.

Different intermediate filaments are:

- made of vimentins. Vimentin intermediate filaments are in general present in mesenchymal cells.
- made of keratin. Keratin is present in general in epithelial cells.
- neurofilaments of neural cells.
- made of lamin, giving structural support to the nuclear envelope.
- made of desmin, play an important role in structural and mechanical support of muscle cells.

Microtubules

Microtubules are hollow cylinders about 23 nm in diameter (lumen = approximately 15 nm in diameter), most commonly comprising 13 protofilaments that, in turn, are polymers of alpha and beta tubulin. They have a very dynamic behavior, binding GTP for polymerization. They are commonly organized by the centrosome.

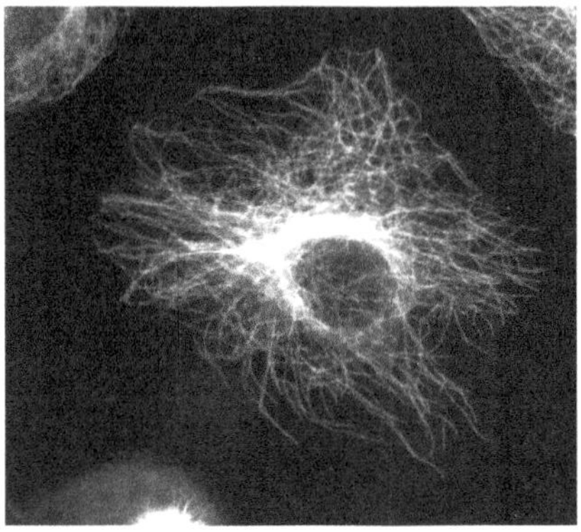

Microtubules in a gel-fixated cell

In nine triplet sets (star-shaped), they form the centrioles, and in nine doublets oriented about two additional microtubules (wheel-shaped), they form cilia and flagella. The latter formation is commonly referred to as a "9+2" arrangement, wherein each doublet is connected to another by the protein dynein. As both flagella and cilia are structural components of the cell, and are maintained by microtubules, they can be considered part of the cytoskeleton.

They play key roles in:

- intracellular transport (associated with dyneins and kinesins, they transport organelles like mitochondria or vesicles).
- the axoneme of cilia and flagella.
- the mitotic spindle.
- synthesis of the cell wall in plants.

Comparison

Cytoskeleton type	Diameter (nm)	Structure	Subunit examples
Microfilaments	6	double helix	actin
Intermediate filaments	10	two anti-parallel helices/ dimers, forming tetramers	• vimentin (mesenchyme) • glial fibrillary acidic protein (glial cells) • neurofilament proteins (neuronal processes) • keratins (epithelial cells) • nuclear lamins

Microtubules	23	protofilaments, in turn consisting of tubulin subunits in complex with stathmin	α- and β-tubulin

Septins

Septins are a group of the highly conserved GTP binding proteins found in eukaryotes. Different septins form protein complexes with each other. These can assemble to filaments and rings. Therefore, septins can be considered part of the cytoskeleton. The function of septins in cells include serving as a localized attachment site for other proteins, and preventing the diffusion of certain molecules from one cell compartment to another. In yeast cells, they build scaffolding to provide structural support during cell division and compartmentalize parts of the cell. Recent research in human cells suggests that septins build cages around bacterial pathogens, immobilizing the harmful microbes and preventing them from invading other cells.

Spectrin

Spectrin is a cytoskeletal protein that lines the intracellular side of the plasma membrane in eukaryotic cells. Spectrin forms pentagonal or hexagonal arrangements, forming a scaffolding and playing an important role in maintenance of plasma membrane integrity and cytoskeletal structure.

Yeast Cytoskeleton

In budding yeast (an important model organism), actin forms cortical patches, actin cables, and a cytokinetic ring and the cap. Cortical patches are discrete actin bodies on the membrane and are important for endocytosis, especially the recycling of glucan synthase which is important for cell wall synthesis. Actin cables are bundles of actin filaments and are involved in the transport of vesicles towards the cap (which contains a number of different proteins to polarize cell growth) and in the positioning of mitochondria. The cytokinetic ring forms and constricts around the site of cell division.

Prokaryotic Cytoskeleton

The cytoskeleton was once thought to be a feature only of eukaryotic cells, but homologues to all the major proteins of the eukaryotic cytoskeleton have been found in prokaryotes. Although the evolutionary relationships are so distant that they are not obvious from protein sequence comparisons alone, the similarity of their three-dimensional structures and similar functions in maintaining cell shape and polarity provides strong evidence that the eukaryotic and prokaryotic cytoskeletons are truly homologous. However, some structures in the bacterial cytoskeleton may not have been identified as of yet.

FtsZ

FtsZ was the first protein of the prokaryotic cytoskeleton to be identified. Like tubulin, FtsZ forms filaments in the presence of guanosine triphosphate (GTP), but these filaments do not group into tubules. During cell division, FtsZ is the first protein to move to the division site, and is essential for recruiting other proteins that synthesize the new cell wall between the dividing cells.

MreB and ParM

Prokaryotic actin-like proteins, such as MreB, are involved in the maintenance of cell shape. All non-spherical bacteria have genes encoding actin-like proteins, and these proteins form a helical network beneath the cell membrane that guides the proteins involved in cell wall biosynthesis.

Some plasmids encode a partitioning system that involves an actin-like protein ParM. Filaments of ParM exhibit dynamic instability, and may partition plasmid DNA into the dividing daughter cells by a mechanism analogous to that used by microtubules during eukaryotic mitosis.

Crescentin

The bacterium *Caulobacter crescentus* contains a third protein, crescentin, that is related to the intermediate filaments of eukaryotic cells. Crescentin is also involved in maintaining cell shape, such as helical and vibrioid forms of bacteria, but the mechanism by which it does this is currently unclear.

Common Features and Differences between Prokaryotes and Eukaryotes

By definition, the cytoskeleton is composed of proteins that can form longitudinal arrays (fibres) in all organisms. These filament forming proteins have been classified into 4 classes. Tubulin-like, actin-like, Walker A cytoskeletal ATPases (WACA-proteins), and intermediate filaments.

Tubulin-like proteins are tubulin in eukaryotes and FtsZ, TubZ, RepX in prokaryotes. Actin-like proteins are actin in eukaryotes and MreB, FtsA in prokaryotes. An example of a WACA-proteins, which are mostly found in prokaryotes, is MinD. Examples for intermediate filaments, which have almost exclusively been found in animals (i.e. eukaryotes) are the lamins, keratins, vimentin, neurofilaments, desmin.

Although tubulin-like proteins share some amino acid sequence similarity, their similarity in protein-fold and the similarity in the GTP binding site is more striking. The same holds true for the actin-like proteins and their structure and ATP binding domain.

Cytoskeletal proteins are usually associated with cell shape, DNA segregation and cell division in prokaryotes and eukaryotes. Which proteins fulfill which task is very different. For example, DNA segregation in all eukaryotes happens through use of tubulin, but in prokaryotes either WACA proteins, actin-like or tubulin-like proteins can be used. Cell division is mediated in eukaryotes by actin, but in prokaryotes usually by tubulin-like (often FtsZ-ring) proteins and sometimes (Crenarchaeota) ESCRT-III, which in eukaryotes still has a role in the last step of division.

Endoskeleton

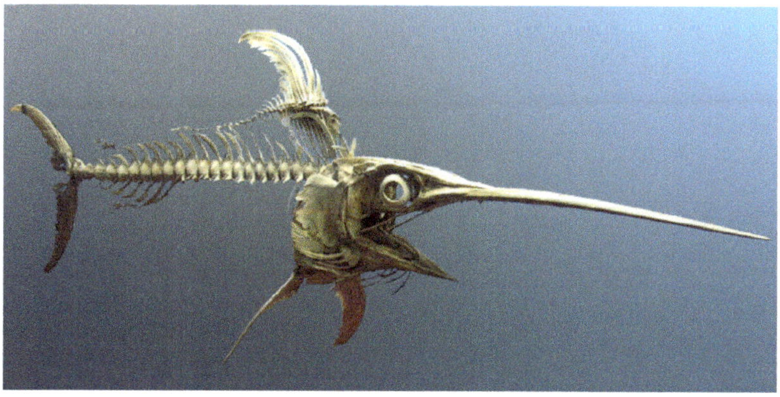

Endoskeleton of a swordfish

An endoskeleton is an internal support structure of an animal, composed of mineralized tissue.

Overview

An endoskeleton is a skeleton that is on the inside of a body. The endoskeleton develops within the skin or in the deeper body tissues. The vertebrate endoskeleton is basically made up of two types of tissues (bone and cartilage). During early embryonic development the endoskeleton is composed of notochord and cartilage. The notochord in most vertebrates is replaced by the vertebral column and cartilage is replaced by bone in most adults. In three phyla and one subclass of animals, endoskeletons of various complexity are found: Chordata, Echinodermata, Porifera, and Coleoidea. An endoskeleton may function purely for support (as in the case of sponges), but often serves as an attachment site for muscle and a mechanism for transmitting muscular forces. A true endoskeleton is derived from mesodermal tissue. Such a skeleton is present in echinoderms and chordates. The poriferan 'skeleton' consists of microscopic calcareous or siliceous spicules or a spongin network. The Coleoidae do not have a true endoskeleton in the evolutionary sense; there, a mollusk exoskeleton evolved into several sorts of internal structure, the "cuttlebone" of cuttlefish being the best-known version. Yet they do have cartilaginous tissue in their body, even if it is not mineralized, especially in the head, where it forms a primitive cranium.The endoskeleton gives shape, support, and protection to the body and provides a means of locomotion.

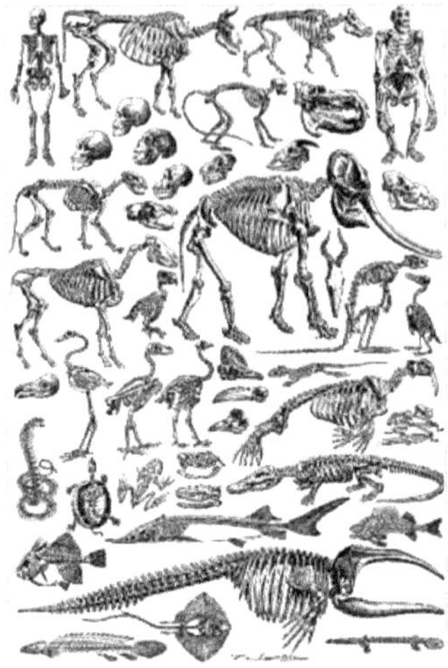

Human Skeleton

The human skeleton is the internal framework of the body. It is composed of around 305 bones at birth – this total decreases to around 206 bones by adulthood after some bones have fused together. The bone mass in the skeleton reaches maximum density around age 21. The human skeleton can be divided into the axial skeleton and the appendicular skeleton. The axial skeleton is formed by the vertebral column, the rib cage, the skull and other associated bones. The appendicular skeleton, which is attached to the axial skeleton, is formed by the shoulder girdle, the pelvic girdle and the bones of the upper and lower limbs.

The human skeleton performs six major functions; support, movement, protection, production of blood cells, storage of minerals, and endocrine regulation.

The human skeleton is not as sexually dimorphic as that of many other primate species, but subtle differences between sexes in the morphology of the skull, dentition, long bones, and pelvis exist. In general, female skeletal elements tend to be smaller and less robust than corresponding male elements within a given population. The human female pelvis is also different from that of males in order to facilitate child birth. Unlike most primates, human males do not have penile bones.

Divisions

Axial Skeleton

The axial skeleton (80 bones) is formed by the vertebral column (32–34 bones; the number of the vertebrae differs from human to human as the lower 2 parts, sacral and coccygeal bone may vary in length), a part of the rib cage (12 pairs of ribs and the sternum), and the skull (22 bones and 7 associated bones).

The upright posture of humans is maintained by the axial skeleton, which transmits the weight from the head, the trunk, and the upper extremities down to the lower extremities at the hip joints. The bones of the spine are supported by many ligaments. The erector spinae muscles are also supporting and are useful for balance.

Appendicular Skeleton

The appendicular skeleton (126 bones) is formed by the pectoral girdles, the upper limbs, the pelvic girdle or pelvis, and the lower limbs. Their functions are to make locomotion possible and to protect the major organs of digestion, excretion and reproduction.

Functions

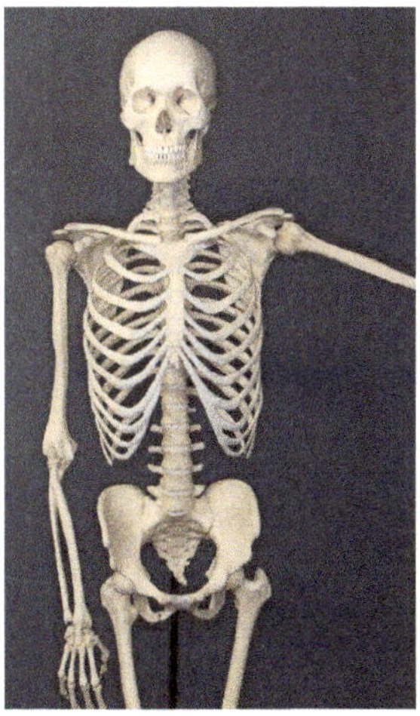

A human skeleton on exhibit at the Museum of Osteology, Oklahoma City, Oklahoma.

The skeleton serves six major functions: support, movement, protection, production of blood cells, storage of minerals and endocrine regulation.

Support

The skeleton provides the framework which supports the body and maintains its shape. The pelvis, associated ligaments and muscles provide a floor for the pelvic structures. Without the rib cages, costal cartilages, and intercostal muscles, the lungs would collapse.

Movement

The joints between bones allow movement, some allowing a wider range of movement than others, e.g. the ball and socket joint allows a greater range of movement than the pivot joint at the neck. Movement is powered by skeletal muscles, which are attached to the skeleton at various sites on bones. Muscles, bones, and joints provide the principal mechanics for movement, all coordinated by the nervous system.

It is believed that the reduction of human bone density in prehistoric times reduced the agility and dexterity of human movement. Shifting from hunting to agriculture has caused human bone density to reduce significantly.

Protection

The skeleton helps to protect our many vital internal organs from being damaged.

- The skull protects the brain
- The vertebrae protect the spinal cord.
- The rib cage, spine, and sternum protect the lungs, heart and major blood vessels.

Blood Cell Production

The skeleton is the site of haematopoiesis, the development of blood cells that takes place in the bone marrow. In children, haematopoiesis occurs primarily in the marrow of the long bones such as the femur and tibia. In adults, it occurs mainly in the pelvis, cranium, vertebrae, and sternum.

Storage

The bone matrix can store calcium and is involved in calcium metabolism, and bone marrow can store iron in ferritin and is involved in iron metabolism. However, bones are not entirely made of calcium, but a mixture of chondroitin sulfate and hydroxyapatite, the latter making up 70% of a bone. Hydroxyapatite is in turn composed of 39.8% of calcium, 41.4% of oxygen, 18.5% of phosphorus, and 0.2% of hydrogen by mass. Chondroitin sulfate is a sugar made up primarily of oxygen and carbon.

Endocrine Regulation

Bone cells release a hormone called osteocalcin, which contributes to the regulation of blood sugar (glucose) and fat deposition. Osteocalcin increases both the insulin secretion and sensitivity, in addition to boosting the number of insulin-producing cells and reducing stores of fat.

Sex Differences

Anatomical differences between human males and females are highly pronounced in some soft tissue areas, but tend to be limited in the skeleton. The human skeleton is not as sexually dimorphic as that of many other primate species, but subtle differences between sexes in the morphology of the skull, dentition, long bones, and pelvis are exhibited across human populations. In general, female skeletal elements tend to be smaller and less robust than corresponding male elements within a given population.

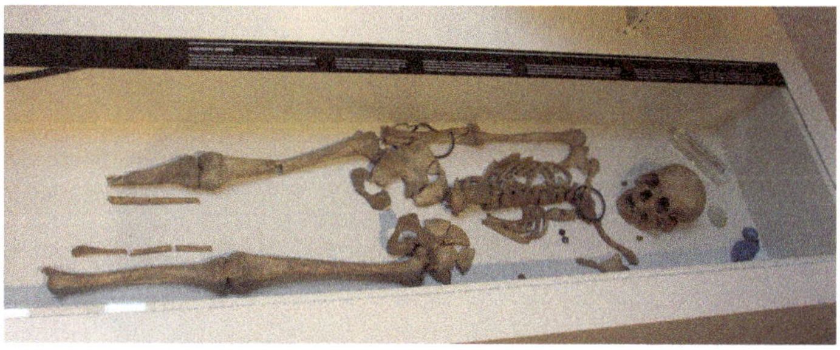

During construction of the York to Scarborough Railway Bridge in 1901, workmen discovered a large stone coffin, close to the River Ouse. Inside was a skeleton, accompanied by an array of unusual and expensive objects. This chance find represents one of the most significant discoveries ever made from Roman York. Study of the skeleton has revealed that it belonged to a woman.

Skull

A variety of gross morphological traits of the human skull demonstrate sexual dimorphism, such as the median nuchal line, mastoid processes, supraorbital margin, supraorbital ridge, and the chin.

Dentition

Human inter-sex dental dimorphism centers on the canine teeth, but it is not nearly as pronounced as in the other great apes.

Long Bones

Long bones are generally larger in males than in females within a given population. Muscle attachment sites on long bones are often more robust in males than in females, reflecting a difference in overall muscle mass and development between sexes. Sexual dimorphism in the long bones is commonly characterized by morphometric or gross morphological analyses.

Pelvis

The human pelvis exhibits greater sexual dimorphism than other bones, specifically in the size and shape of the pelvic cavity, ilia, greater sciatic notches, and the sub-pubic angle. The Phenice method is commonly used to determine the sex of an unidentified human skeleton by anthropologists with 96% to 100% accuracy in some populations.

Women's pelvises are wider in the pelvic inlet and are wider throughout the pelvis to allow for child birth. The sacrum in the women's pelvis is curved in wards to allow the child to have a "funnel" to assist in the child's pathway from the uterus to the birth canal.

Clinical Significance

There are many classified skeletal disorders. One of the most common is osteoporosis. Also common is scoliosis, a side-to-side curve in the back or spine, often creating a pronounced "C" or "S" shape when viewed on an x-ray of the spine. This condition is most apparent during adolescence, and is most common with females.

Arthritis

Arthritis is a disorder of the joints. It involves inflammation of one or more joints. When affected by arthritis, the joint or joints affected may be painful to move, may move in unusual directions or may be immobile completely. The symptoms of arthritis will vary differently between types of arthritis. The most common form of arthritis: Osteoarthritis can affect both the larger and smaller joints of the human skeleton. The cartilage in the affected joints will degrade, soften and wear away. This decreases the mobility of the joints and decreases the space between bones where cartilage should be.

Osteoporosis

Osteoporosis is a disease of bone where there is reduced bone mineral density, increasing the likelihood of fractures. Osteoporosis is defined by the World Health Organization in women as a bone mineral density 2.5 standard deviations below peak bone mass, relative to the age and sex-matched average, as measured by Dual energy X-ray absorptiometry, with the term "established osteoporosis" including the presence of a fragility fracture. Osteoporosis is most common in women after menopause, when it is called "postmenopausal osteoporosis", but may develop in men and premenopausal women in the presence of particular hormonal disorders and other chronic diseases or as a result of smoking and medications, specifically glucocorticoids. Osteoporosis usually has no symptoms until a fracture occurs. For this reason, DEXA scans are often done in people with one or more risk factors, who have developed osteoporosis and be at risk of fracture.

Osteoporosis treatment includes advice to stop smoking, decrease alcohol consumption, exercise regularly, and have a healthy diet. Calcium supplements may also be advised, as may Vitamin D. When medication is used, it may include bisphosphonates, Strontium ranelate, and osteoporosis may be one factor considered when commencing Hormone replacement therapy.

History

The study of human bones probably started in ancient Greece under Ptolemaic kings due to their link to Egypt. Herophilos, through his work by studying dissected human corpses in Alexandria is credited to be the pioneer of the field. His works are lost but are often cited by notable perons in the field such as Galen and Rufus of Ephesus. Galen himself did little dissection though and relied on the work of others like Marinus of Alexandria, as well as his own observations of gladiator cadavers and animals. According to Katherine Park, in medieval Europe dissection continued to be practiced, contrary to the popular understanding that such practices are taboo and thus completely banned. The practice of *holy autopsy,* such as in the case of Clare of Montefalco further supports the claim. Alexandria continued as a center of anatomy under Islamic rule, with Ibn Zuhr a notable figure. Chinese understandings are divergent, as the closest corresponding concept in the medicinal system seem to be the meridians, although given that Hua Tuo regularly performs surgery, there must be some distance between medical theory and actual understanding.

The Renaissance

Leonardo Da Vinci, among his many talents also contributed to the study of the skeleton, albeit unpublished in his time. Many artists, Antonio Pollaiuolo being the first, performed dissections for better understanding of the body, although they concentrated mostly on the muscles. Vesalius, regarded as the founder of modern anatomy authored the book *De humani corporis fabrica* ,which contained many illustrations of the skeleton and other body parts, correcting some theories dating from Galen, such as the lower jaw being a single bone instead of two. Various other figures like Alessandro Achillini also contributed to the further understanding of the skeleton.

Human Musculoskeletal System

The human musculoskeletal system (also known as the locomotor system, and previously the activity system) is an organ system that gives humans the ability to move using their muscular and skeletal systems. The musculoskeletal system provides form, support, stability, and movement to the body.

It is made up of the bones of the skeleton, muscles, cartilage, tendons, ligaments, joints, and other connective tissue that supports and binds tissues and organs together. The musculoskeletal system's primary functions include supporting the body, allowing motion, and protecting vital organs. The skeletal portion of the system serves as the main storage system for calcium and phosphorus and contains critical components of the hematopoietic system.

This system describes how bones are connected to other bones and muscle fibers via connective tissue such as tendons and ligaments. The bones provide stability to the body. Muscles keep bones in place and also play a role in the movement of bones. To allow motion, different bones are connected by joints. Cartilage prevents the bone ends from rubbing directly onto each other. Muscles contract to move the bone attached at the joint.

There are, however, diseases and disorders that may adversely affect the function and overall effectiveness of the system. These diseases can be difficult to diagnose due to the close relation of the musculoskeletal system to other internal systems. The musculoskeletal system refers to the system having its muscles attached to an internal skeletal system and is necessary for humans to move to a more favorable position. Complex issues and injuries involving the musculoskeletal system are usually handled by a physiatrist (specialist in physical medicine and rehabilitation) or an orthopaedic surgeon.

Subsystems

Skeletal

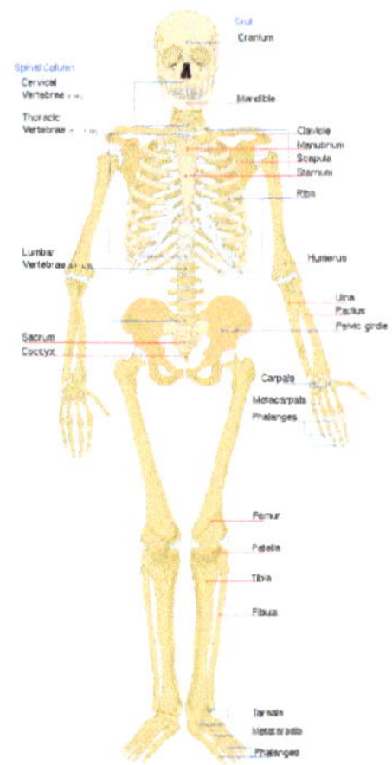

Front view of a skeleton of an adult human

The skeletal system serves many important functions; it provides the shape and form for the body, support and protection, allows bodily movement, produces blood for the body, and stores minerals. The number of bones in the human skeletal system is a controversial topic. Humans are born with over 300 bones; however, many bones fuse together between birth and maturity. As a result, an average adult skeleton consists of 206 bones. The number of bones varies according to the method used to derive the count. While some consider certain structures to be a single bone with multiple parts, others may see it as a single part with multiple bones. There are five general classifications of bones. These are long bones, short bones, flat bones, irregular bones, and sesamoid bones. The human skeleton is composed of both fused and individual bones supported by ligaments, tendons, muscles and cartilage. It is a complex structure with two distinct divisions; the axial skeleton, which includes the vertebral column, and the appendicular skeleton.

Function

The skeletal system serves as a framework for tissues and organs to attach themselves to. This system acts as a protective structure for vital organs. Major examples of this are the brain being protected by the skull and the lungs being protected by the rib cage.

Located in long bones are two distinctions of bone marrow (yellow and red). The yellow marrow has fatty connective tissue and is found in the marrow cavity. During starvation, the body uses the fat in yellow marrow for energy. The red marrow of some bones is an important site for blood cell production, approximately 2.6 million red blood cells per second in order to replace existing cells that have been destroyed by the liver. Here all erythrocytes, platelets, and most leukocytes form in adults. From the red marrow, erythrocytes, platelets, and leukocytes migrate to the blood to do their special tasks.

Another function of bones is the storage of certain minerals. Calcium and phosphorus are among the main minerals being stored. The importance of this storage "device" helps to regulate mineral balance in the bloodstream. When the fluctuation of minerals is high, these minerals are stored in bone; when it is low it will be withdrawn from the bone.

Muscular

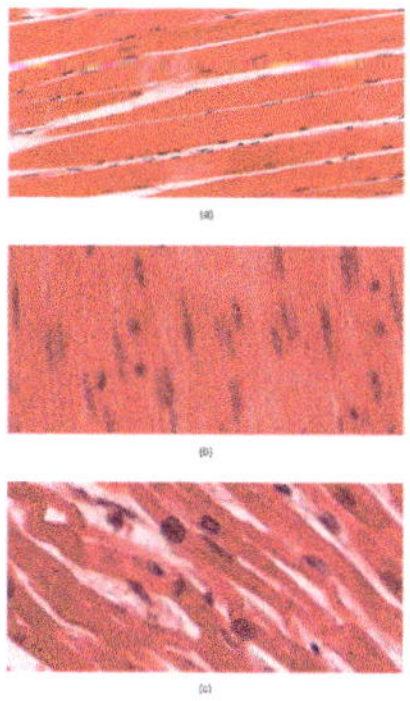

The body contains three types of muscle tissue: (a) skeletal muscle, (b) smooth muscle, and (c) cardiac muscle.

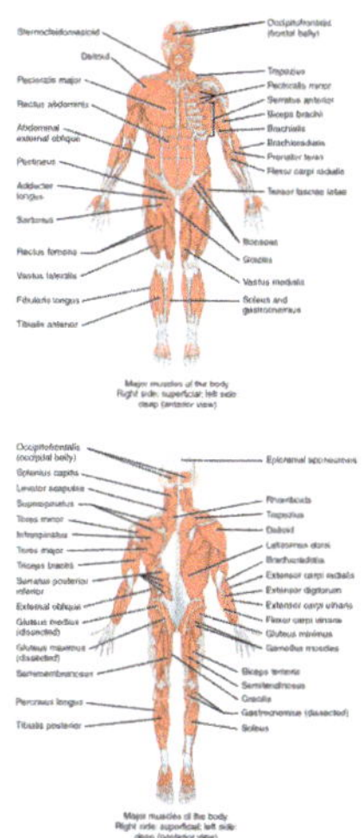

On the anterior and posterior views of the muscular system above, superficial muscles (those at the surface) are shown on the right side of the body while deep muscles (those underneath the superficial muscles) are shown on the left half of the body. For the legs, superficial muscles are shown in the anterior view while the posterior view shows both superficial and deep muscles.

There are three types of muscles—cardiac, skeletal, and smooth. Smooth muscles are used to control the flow of substances within the lumens of hollow organs, and are not consciously controlled. Skeletal and cardiac muscles have striations that are visible under a microscope due to the components within their cells. Only skeletal and smooth muscles are part of the musculoskeletal system and only the skeletal muscles can move the body. Cardiac muscles are found in the heart and are used only to circulate blood; like the smooth muscles, these muscles are not under conscious control. Skeletal muscles are attached to bones and arranged in opposing groups around joints. Muscles are innervated, to communicate nervous energy to, by nerves, which conduct electrical currents from the central nervous system and cause the muscles to contract.

Contraction Initiation

In mammals, when a muscle contracts, a series of reactions occur. Muscle contraction is stimulated by the motor neuron sending a message to the muscles from the somatic nervous system. Depolarization of the motor neuron results in neurotransmitters being released from the nerve terminal. The space between the nerve terminal and the muscle cell is called the neuromuscular junction. These neurotransmitters diffuse across the synapse and bind to specific receptor sites on the cell membrane of the muscle fiber. When enough receptors are stimulated, an action potential is generated and the permeability of the sarcolemma is altered. This process is known as initiation.

Tendons

A tendon is a tough, flexible band of fibrous connective tissue that connects muscles to bones. The extra-cellular connective tissue between muscle fibers binds to tendons at the distal and proximal ends, and the tendon binds to the periosteum of individual bones at the muscle's origin and insertion. As muscles contract, tendons transmit the forces to the relatively rigid bones, pulling on them and causing movement. Tendons can stretch substantially, allowing them to function as springs during locomotion, thereby saving energy.

Joints, Ligaments and Bursae

Joints

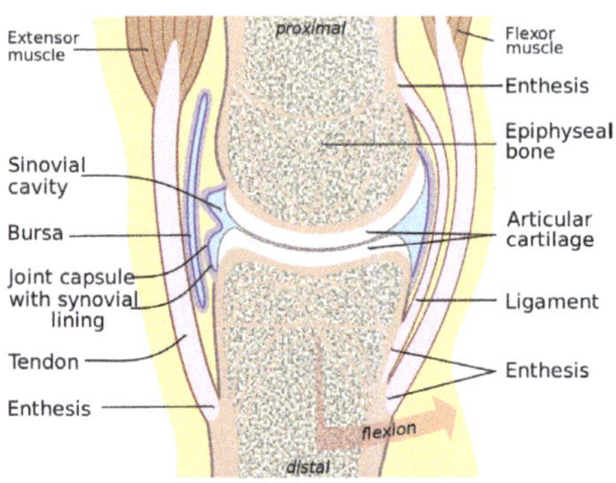

Human synovial joint composition

Joints are structures that connect individual bones and may allow bones to move against each other to cause movement. There are two divisions of joints, diarthroses which allow extensive mobility between two or more articular heads, and false joints or synarthroses, joints that are immovable, that allow little or no movement and are predominantly fibrous. Synovial joints, joints that are not directly joined, are lubricated by a solution called synovial fluid that is produced by the synovial membranes. This fluid lowers the friction between the articular surfaces and is kept within an articular capsule, binding the joint with its taut tissue.

Ligaments

A ligament is a small band of dense, white, fibrous elastic tissue. Ligaments connect the ends of bones together in order to form a joint. Most ligaments limit dislocation, or prevent certain movements that may cause breaks. Since they are only elastic they increasingly lengthen when under pressure. When this occurs the ligament may be susceptible to break resulting in an unstable joint.

Ligaments may also restrict some actions: movements such as hyper extension and hyper flexion are restricted by ligaments to an extent. Also ligaments prevent certain directional movement.

Bursae

A bursa is a small fluid-filled sac made of white fibrous tissue and lined with synovial membrane. Bursa may also be formed by a synovial membrane that extends outside of the joint capsule. It provides a cushion between bones and tendons and/or muscles around a joint; bursa are filled with synovial fluid and are found around almost every major joint of the body.

Clinical Significance

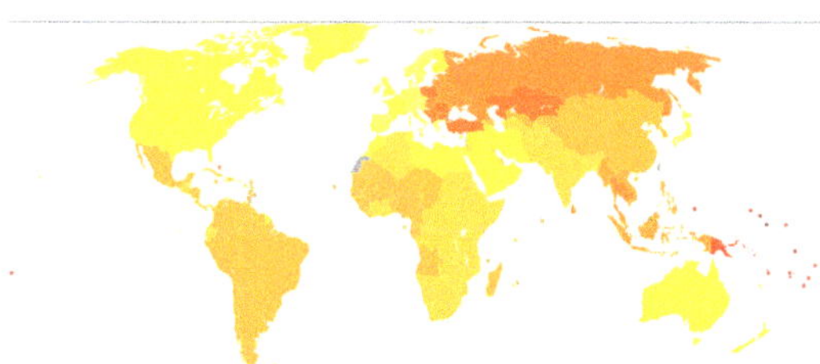

Disability-adjusted life year for musculoskeletal diseases per 100,000 inhabitants in 2004.

- no data
- less than 400
- 400-450
- 450-500
- 500-550
- 550-600
- 600-650
- 650-700
- 700-850
- 850-900
- 900-925
- 925-950
- more than 950

Because many other body systems, including the vascular, nervous, and integumentary systems, are interrelated, disorders of one of these systems may also affect the musculoskeletal system and complicate the diagnosis of the disorder's origin. Diseases of the musculoskeletal system mostly encompass functional disorders or motion discrepancies; the level of impairment depends specifically on the problem and its severity. In a study of hospitalizations in the United States, the most common inpatient OR procedures in 2012 involved the musculoskeletal system: knee arthroplasty, laminectomy, hip replacement, and spinal fusion.

Articular (of or pertaining to the joints) disorders are the most common. However, also among the diagnoses are: primary muscular diseases, neurologic (related to the medical science that deals with the nervous system and disorders affecting it) deficits, toxins, endocrine abnormalities, metabolic disorders, infectious diseases, blood and vascular disorders, and nutritional imbalances.

Disorders of muscles from another body system can bring about irregularities such as: impairment of ocular motion and control, respiratory dysfunction, and bladder malfunction. Complete paralysis, paresis, or ataxia may be caused by primary muscular dysfunctions of infectious or toxic origin; however, the primary disorder is usually related to the nervous system, with the muscular system acting as the effector organ, an organ capable of responding to a stimulus, especially a nerve impulse.

One understated disorder that begins during pregnancy is Pelvic girdle pain, it is complex and multi-factorial and likely to be also represented by a series of sub-groups driven by pain varying from peripheral or central nervous system, altered laxity/stiffness of muscles, laxity to injury of tendinous/ligamentous structures to 'mal-adaptive' body mechanics.

Muscle

Muscle is a soft tissue found in most animals. Muscle cells contain protein filaments of actin and myosin that slide past one another, producing a contraction that changes both the length and the shape of the cell. Muscles function to produce force and motion. They are primarily responsible for maintaining and changing posture, locomotion, as well as movement of internal organs, such as the contraction of the heart and the movement of food through the digestive system via peristalsis.

Muscle tissues are derived from the mesodermal layer of embryonic germ cells in a process known as myogenesis. There are three types of muscle, skeletal or striated, cardiac, and smooth. Muscle action can be classified as being either voluntary or involuntary. Cardiac and smooth muscles contract without conscious thought and are termed involuntary, whereas the skeletal muscles contract upon command. Skeletal muscles in turn can be divided into fast and slow twitch fibers.

Muscles are predominantly powered by the oxidation of fats and carbohydrates, but anaerobic chemical reactions are also used, particularly by fast twitch fibers. These chemical reactions produce adenosine triphosphate (ATP) molecules that are used to power the movement of the myosin heads.

The term muscle is derived from the Latin *musculus* meaning "little mouse" perhaps because of the shape of certain muscles or because contracting muscles look like mice moving under the skin.

Anatomy

The anatomy of muscles includes gross anatomy, which comprises all the muscles of an organism, and microanatomy, which comprises the structures of a single muscle.

Types of Tissue

Muscle tissue is a soft tissue, and is one of the four fundamental types of tissue present in animals. There are three types of muscle tissue recognized in vertebrates:

- Skeletal muscle or "voluntary muscle" is anchored by tendons (or by aponeuroses at a few places) to bone and is used to effect skeletal movement such as locomotion and in maintaining posture. Though this postural control is generally maintained as an unconscious reflex, the muscles responsible react to conscious control like non-postural muscles. An average adult male is made up of 42% of skeletal muscle and an average adult female is made up of 36% (as a percentage of body mass).
- Smooth muscle or "involuntary muscle" is found within the walls of organs and structures such as the esophagus, stomach, intestines, bronchi, uterus, urethra, bladder, blood vessels, and the arrector pili in the skin (in which it controls erection of body hair). Unlike skeletal muscle, smooth muscle is not under conscious control.
- Cardiac muscle (myocardium), is also an "involuntary muscle" but is more akin in structure to skeletal muscle, and is found only in the heart.

Cardiac and skeletal muscles are "striated" in that they contain sarcomeres that are packed into highly regular arrangements of bundles; the myofibrils of smooth muscle cells are not arranged in sarcomeres and so are not striated. While the sarcomeres in skeletal muscles are arranged in regular, parallel bundles, cardiac muscle sarcomeres connect at branching, irregular angles (called intercalated discs). Striated muscle contracts and relaxes in short, intense bursts, whereas smooth muscle sustains longer or even near-permanent contractions.

Skeletal (voluntary) muscle is further divided into two broad types: *slow twitch* and *fast twitch*:

- Type I, slow twitch, or "red" muscle, is dense with capillaries and is rich in mitochondria and myoglobin, giving the muscle tissue its characteristic red color. It can carry more oxygen and sustain aerobic activity using fats or carbohydrates as fuel. Slow twitch fibers contract for long periods of time but with little force.
- Type II, fast twitch muscle, has three major subtypes (IIa, IIx, and IIb) that vary in both contractile speed and force generated. Fast twitch fibers contract quickly and powerfully but fatigue very rapidly, sustaining only short, anaerobic bursts of activity before muscle contraction becomes painful. They contribute most to muscle strength and have greater potential for increase in mass. Type IIb is anaerobic, glycolytic, "white" muscle that is least dense in mitochondria and myoglobin. In small animals (e.g., rodents) this is the major fast muscle type, explaining the pale color of their flesh.

The density of mammalian skeletal muscle tissue is about 1.06 kg/liter. This can be contrasted with the density of adipose tissue (fat), which is 0.9196 kg/liter. This makes muscle tissue approximately 15% denser than fat tissue.

Histogenesis

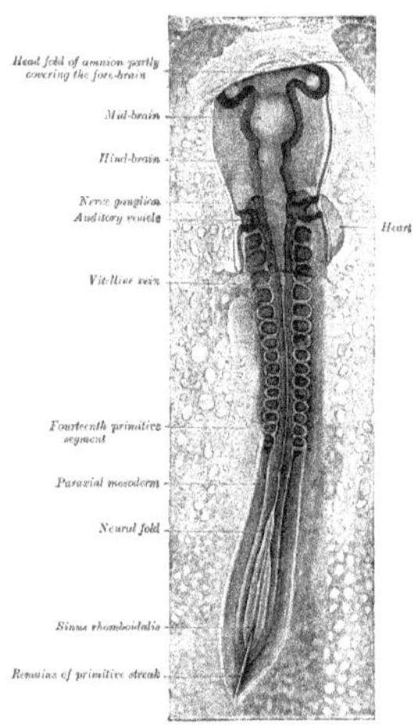

A chicken embryo, showing the paraxial mesoderm on both sides of the neural fold. The anterior (forward) portion has begun to form somites (labeled "primitive segments").

All muscles are derived from paraxial mesoderm. The paraxial mesoderm is divided along the embryo's length into somites, corresponding to the segmentation of the body (most obviously seen in the vertebral column. Each somite has 3 divisions, sclerotome (which forms vertebrae), dermatome (which forms skin), and myotome (which forms muscle). The myotome is divided into two sections, the epimere and hypomere, which form epaxial and hypaxial muscles, respectively. The only epaxial muscles in humans are the erector spinae and small intervertebral muscles, and are innervated by the dorsal rami of the spinal nerves. All other muscles, including those of the limbs are hypaxial, and inervated by the ventral rami of the spinal nerves.

During development, myoblasts (muscle progenitor cells) either remain in the somite to form muscles associated with the vertebral column or migrate out into the body to form all other muscles. Myoblast migration is preceded by the formation of connective tissue frameworks, usually formed from the somatic lateral plate mesoderm. Myoblasts follow chemical signals to the appropriate locations, where they fuse into elongate skeletal muscle cells.

Microanatomy

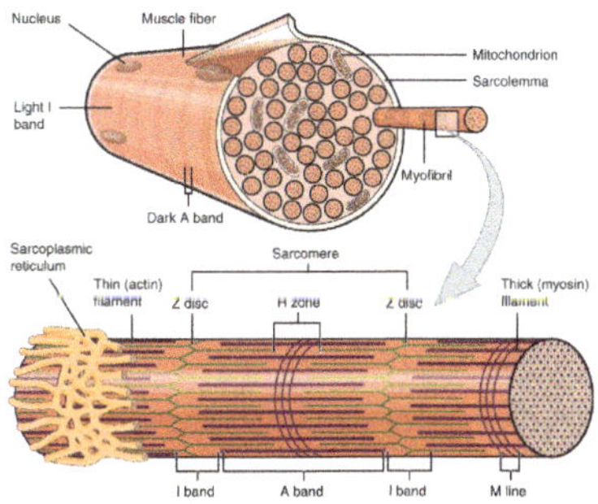

A skeletal muscle fiber is surrounded by a plasma membrane called the sarcolemma, which contains sarcoplasm, the cytoplasm of muscle cells. A muscle fiber is composed of many fibrils, which give the cell its striated appearance.

Skeletal muscles are sheathed by a tough layer of connective tissue called the epimysium. The epimysium anchors muscle tissue to tendons at each end, where the epimysium becomes thicker and collagenous. It also protects muscles from friction against other muscles and bones. Within the epimysium are multiple bundles called fascicles, each of which contains 10 to 100 or more muscle fibers collectively sheathed by a perimysium. Besides surrounding each fascicle, the perimysium is a pathway for nerves and the flow of blood within the muscle. The threadlike muscle fibers are the individual muscle cells (myocytes), and each cell is encased within its own endomysium of collagen fibers. Thus, the overall muscle consists of fibers (cells) that are bundled into fascicles, which are themselves grouped together to form muscles. At each level of bundling, a collagenous membrane surrounds the bundle, and these membranes support muscle function both by resisting passive stretching of the tissue and by distributing forces applied to the muscle. Scattered throughout the muscles are muscle spindles that provide sensory feedback information to the central nervous system. (This grouping structure is analogous to the organization of nerves which uses epineurium, perineurium, and endoneurium).

This same bundles-within-bundles structure is replicated within the muscle cells. Within the cells of the muscle are myofibrils, which themselves are bundles of protein filaments. The term "myofibril" should not be confused with "myofiber", which is a simply another name for a muscle cell. Myofibrils are complex strands of several kinds of protein filaments organized together into repeating units called sarcomeres. The striated appearance of both skeletal and cardiac muscle results from the regular pattern of sarcomeres within their cells. Although both of these types of muscle contain sarcomeres, the fibers in cardiac muscle are typically branched to form a network. Cardiac muscle fibers are interconnected by intercalated discs, giving that tissue the appearance of a syncytium.

The filaments in a sarcomere are composed of actin and myosin.

Gross Anatomy

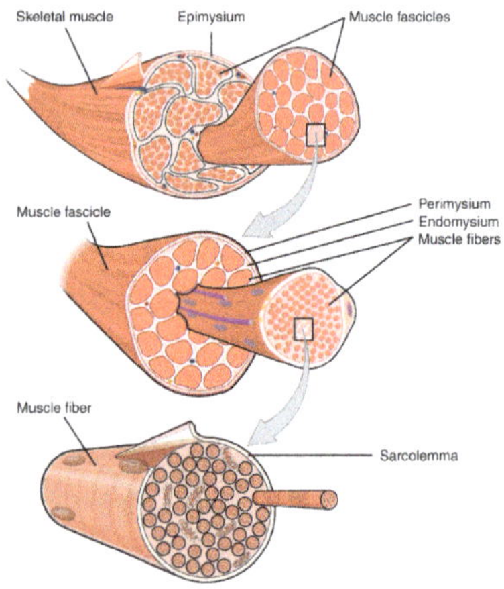

Bundles of muscle fibers, called fascicles, are covered by the perimysium. Muscle fibers are covered by the endomysium.

The gross anatomy of a muscle is the most important indicator of its role in the body. There is an important distinction seen between pennate muscles and other muscles. In most muscles, all the fibers are oriented in the same direction, running in a line from the origin to the insertion. However, In pennate muscles, the individual fibers are oriented at an angle relative to the line of action, attaching to the origin and insertion tendons at each end. Because the contracting fibers are pulling at an angle to the overall action of the muscle, the change in length is smaller, but this same orientation allows for more fibers (thus more force) in a muscle of a given size. Pennate muscles are usually found where their length change is less important than maximum force, such as the rectus femoris.

Skeletal muscle is arranged in discrete muscles, an example of which is the *biceps brachii* (biceps). The tough, fibrous epimysium of skeletal muscle is both connected to and continuous with the tendons. In turn, the tendons connect to the periosteum layer surrounding the bones, permitting the transfer of force from the muscles to the skeleton. Together, these fibrous layers, along with tendons and ligaments, constitute the deep fascia of the body.

Muscular System

The muscular system consists of all the muscles present in a single body. There are approximately 650 skeletal muscles in the human body, but an exact number is difficult to define. The difficulty lies partly in the fact that different sources group the muscles differently and partly in that some muscles, such as palmaris longus, are not always present.

A muscular *slip* is a narrow length of muscle that acts to augment a larger muscle or muscles.

The muscular system is one component of the musculoskeletal system, which includes not only the muscles but also the bones, joints, tendons, and other structures that permit movement.

Physiology

The three types of muscle (skeletal, cardiac and smooth) have significant differences. However, all three use the movement of actin against myosin to create contraction. In skeletal muscle, contraction is stimulated by electrical impulses transmitted by the nerves, the motoneurons (motor nerves) in particular. Cardiac and smooth muscle contractions are stimulated by internal pacemaker cells which regularly contract, and propagate contractions to other muscle cells they are in contact with. All skeletal muscle and many smooth muscle contractions are facilitated by the neurotransmitter acetylcholine.

Function

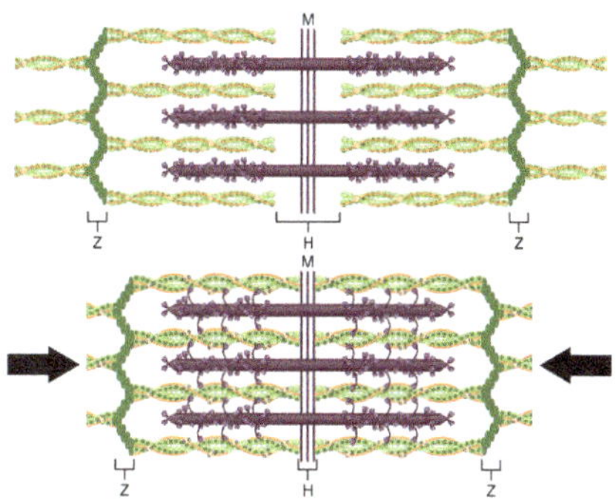

When a sarcomere contracts, the Z lines move closer together, and the I band becomes smaller. The A band stays the same width. At full contraction, the thin and thick filaments overlap.

The action a muscle generates is determined by the origin and insertion locations. The cross-sectional area of a muscle (rather than volume or length) determines the amount of force it can generate by defining the number of "sarcomeres" which can operate in parallel. Each skeletal muscle contains long units called myofibrils, and each myofibril is a chain of sarcomeres. Since contraction occurs at the same time for all connected sarcomeres in a muscles cell, these chains of sarcomeres shorten together, thus shortening the muscle fiber, resulting in overall length change. The amount of force applied to the external environment is determined by lever mechanics, specifically the ratio of in-lever to out-lever. For example, moving the insertion point of the biceps more distally on the radius (farther from the joint of rotation) would increase the force generated during flexion (and, as a result, the maximum weight lifted in this movement), but decrease the maximum speed of flexion. Moving the insertion point proximally (closer to the joint of rotation) would result in decreased force but increased velocity. This can be most easily seen by comparing the limb of a mole to a horse - in the former, the insertion point is positioned to maximize force (for digging), while in the latter, the insertion point is positioned to maximize speed (for running).

Energy Consumption

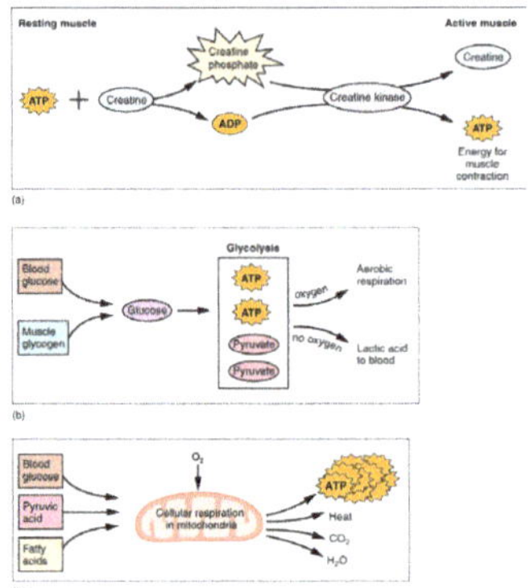

(a) Some ATP is stored in a resting muscle. As contraction starts, it is used up in seconds. More ATP is generated from creatine phosphate for about 15 seconds. (b) Each glucose molecule produces two ATP and two molecules of pyruvic acid, which can be used in aerobic respiration or converted to lactic acid. If oxygen is not available, pyruvic acid is converted to lactic acid, which may contribute to muscle fatigue. This occurs during strenuous exercise when high amounts of energy are needed but oxygen cannot be sufficiently delivered to muscle. (c) Aerobic respiration is the breakdown of glucose in the presence of oxygen (O2) to produce carbon dioxide, water, and ATP. Approximately 95 percent of the ATP required for resting or moderately active muscles is provided by aerobic respiration, which takes place in mitochondria.

Muscular activity accounts for much of the body's energy consumption. All muscle cells produce adenosine triphosphate (ATP) molecules which are used to power the movement of the myosin heads. Muscles have a short-term store of energy in the form of creatine phosphate which is generated from ATP and can regenerate ATP when needed with creatine kinase. Muscles also keep a storage form of glucose in the form of glycogen. Glycogen can be rapidly converted to glucose when energy is required for sustained, powerful contractions. Within the voluntary skeletal muscles, the glucose molecule can be metabolized anaerobically in a process called glycolysis which produces two ATP and two lactic acid molecules in the process (in aerobic conditions, lactate is not formed; instead pyruvate is formed and transmitted through the citric acid cycle). Muscle cells also contain globules of fat, which are used for energy during aerobic exercise. The aerobic energy systems take longer to produce the ATP and reach peak efficiency, and requires many more biochemical steps, but produces significantly more ATP than anaerobic glycolysis. Cardiac muscle on the other hand, can readily consume any of the three macronutrients (protein, glucose and fat) aerobically without a 'warm up' period and always extracts the maximum ATP yield from any molecule involved. The heart, liver and red blood cells will also consume lactic acid produced and excreted by skeletal muscles during exercise.

At rest, skeletal muscle consumes 54.4 kJ/kg (13.0 kcal/kg) per day. This is larger than adipose tissue (fat) at 18.8 kJ/kg (4.5 kcal/kg), and bone at 9.6 kJ/kg (2.3 kcal/kg).

Nervous Control

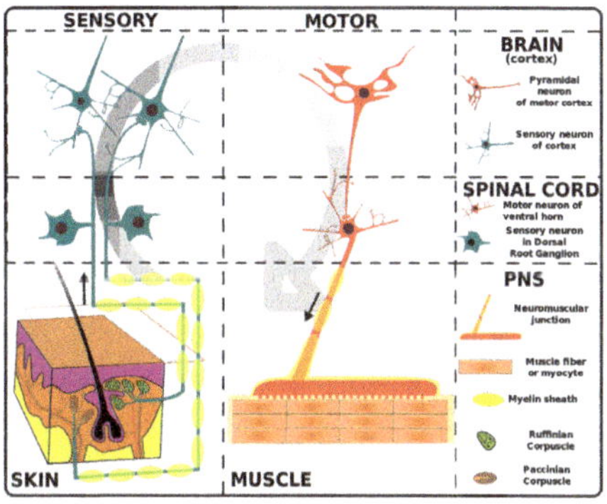

Simplified schema of basic nervous system function. Signals are picked up by sensory receptors and sent to the spinal cord and brain via the afferent leg of the peripheral nervous system, whereupon processing occurs that results in signals sent back to the spinal cord and then out to motor neurons via the efferent leg.

Efferent Leg

The efferent leg of the peripheral nervous system is responsible for conveying commands to the muscles and glands, and is ultimately responsible for voluntary movement. Nerves move muscles in response to voluntary and autonomic (involuntary) signals from the brain. Deep muscles, superficial muscles, muscles of the face and internal muscles all correspond with dedicated regions in the primary motor cortex of the brain, directly anterior to the central sulcus that divides the frontal and parietal lobes.

In addition, muscles react to reflexive nerve stimuli that do not always send signals all the way to the brain. In this case, the signal from the afferent fiber does not reach the brain, but produces the reflexive movement by direct connections with the efferent nerves in the spine. However, the majority of muscle activity is volitional, and the result of complex interactions between various areas of the brain.

Nerves that control skeletal muscles in mammals correspond with neuron groups along the primary motor cortex of the brain's cerebral cortex. Commands are routed though the basal ganglia and are modified by input from the cerebellum before being relayed through the pyramidal tract to the spinal cord and from there to the motor end plate at the muscles. Along the way, feedback, such as that of the extrapyramidal system contribute signals to influence muscle tone and response.

Deeper muscles such as those involved in posture often are controlled from nuclei in the brain stem and basal ganglia.

Afferent Leg

The afferent leg of the peripheral nervous system is responsible for conveying sensory information to the brain, primarily from the sense organs like the skin. In the muscles, the muscle spindles convey information about the degree of muscle length and stretch to the central nervous system to assist in maintaining posture and joint position. The sense of where our bodies are in space is called proprioception, the perception of body awareness. More easily demonstrated than explained, proprioception is the "unconscious" awareness of where the various regions of the body are located at any one time. This can be demonstrated by anyone closing their eyes and waving their hand around. Assuming proper proprioceptive function, at no time will the person lose awareness of where the hand actually is, even though it is not being detected by any of the other senses.

Several areas in the brain coordinate movement and position with the feedback information gained from proprioception. The cerebellum and red nucleus in particular continuously sample position against movement and make minor corrections to assure smooth motion.

Efficiency

The efficiency of human muscle has been measured (in the context of rowing and cycling) at 18% to 26%. The efficiency is defined as the ratio of mechanical work output to the total metabolic cost, as can be calculated from oxygen consumption. This low efficiency is the result of about 40% efficiency of generating ATP from food energy, losses in converting energy from ATP into mechanical work inside the muscle, and mechanical losses inside the body. The latter two losses are dependent on the type of exercise and the type of muscle fibers being used (fast-twitch or slow-twitch). For an overall efficiency of 20 percent, one watt of mechanical power is equivalent to 4.3 kcal per hour. For example, one manufacturer of rowing equipment calibrates its rowing ergometer to count burned calories as equal to four times the actual mechanical work, plus 300 kcal per hour, this amounts to about 20 percent efficiency at 250 watts of mechanical output. The mechanical energy output of a cyclic contraction can depend upon many factors, including activation timing, muscle strain trajectory, and rates of force rise & decay. These can be synthesized experimentally using work loop analysis.

Strength

A display of "strength" (e.g. lifting a weight) is a result of three factors that overlap: physiological strength (muscle size, cross sectional area, available crossbridging, responses to training), neurological strength (how strong or weak is the signal that tells the muscle to contract), and mechanical strength (muscle's force angle on the lever, moment arm length, joint capabilities).

Physiological Strength

Grading of muscle strength	
Grade 0	No contraction
Grade 1	Trace of contraction, but no movement at the joint
Grade 2	Movement at the joint with gravity eliminated
Grade 3	Movement against gravity, but not against added resistance
Grade 4	Movement against external resistance, but less than normal
Grade 5	Normal strength

Vertebrate muscle typically produces approximately 25–33 N (5.6–7.4 lb_f) of force per square centimeter of muscle cross-sectional area when isometric and at optimal length. Some invertebrate muscles, such as in crab claws, have much longer sarcomeres than vertebrates, resulting in many more sites for actin and myosin to bind and thus much greater force per square centimeter at the cost of much slower speed. The force generated by a contraction can be measured non-invasively using either mechanomyography or phonomyography, be measured in vivo using tendon strain (if a prominent tendon is present), or be measured directly using more invasive methods.

The strength of any given muscle, in terms of force exerted on the skeleton, depends upon length, shortening speed, cross sectional area, pennation, sarcomere length, myosin isoforms, and neural activation of motor units. Significant reductions in muscle strength can indicate underlying pathology, with the chart at right used as a guide.

The "Strongest" Human Muscle

Since three factors affect muscular strength simultaneously and muscles never work individually, it is misleading to compare strength in individual muscles, and state that one is the "strongest". But below are several muscles whose strength is noteworthy for different reasons.

- In ordinary parlance, muscular "strength" usually refers to the ability to exert a force on an external object—for example, lifting a weight. By this definition, the masseter or jaw muscle is the strongest. The 1992 Guinness Book of Records records the achievement of a bite strength of 4,337 N (975 lb_f) for 2 seconds. What distinguishes the masseter is not anything special about the muscle itself, but its advantage in working against a much shorter lever arm than other muscles.
- If "strength" refers to the force exerted by the muscle itself, e.g., on the place where it inserts into a bone, then the strongest muscles are those with the largest cross-sectional area. This is because the tension exerted by an individual skeletal muscle fiber does not vary much. Each fiber can exert a force on the

order of 0.3 micronewton. By this definition, the strongest muscle of the body is usually said to be the quadriceps femoris or the gluteus maximus.

- Because muscle strength is determined by cross-sectional area, a shorter muscle will be stronger "pound for pound" (i.e., by weight) than a longer muscle of the same cross-sectional area. The myometrial layer of the uterus may be the strongest muscle by weight in the female human body. At the time when an infant is delivered, the entire human uterus weighs about 1.1 kg (40 oz). During childbirth, the uterus exerts 100 to 400 N (25 to 100 lbf) of downward force with each contraction.
- The external muscles of the eye are conspicuously large and strong in relation to the small size and weight of the eyeball. It is frequently said that they are "the strongest muscles for the job they have to do" and are sometimes claimed to be "100 times stronger than they need to be." However, eye movements (particularly saccades used on facial scanning and reading) do require high speed movements, and eye muscles are exercised nightly during rapid eye movement sleep.
- The statement that "the tongue is the strongest muscle in the body" appears frequently in lists of surprising facts, but it is difficult to find any definition of "strength" that would make this statement true. The tongue consists of eight muscles, not one.
- The heart has a claim to being the muscle that performs the largest quantity of physical work in the course of a lifetime. Estimates of the power output of the human heart range from 1 to 5 watts. This is much less than the maximum power output of other muscles; for example, the quadriceps can produce over 100 watts, but only for a few minutes. The heart does its work continuously over an entire lifetime without pause, and thus does "outwork" other muscles. An output of one watt continuously for eighty years yields a total work output of two and a half gigajoules.

Health

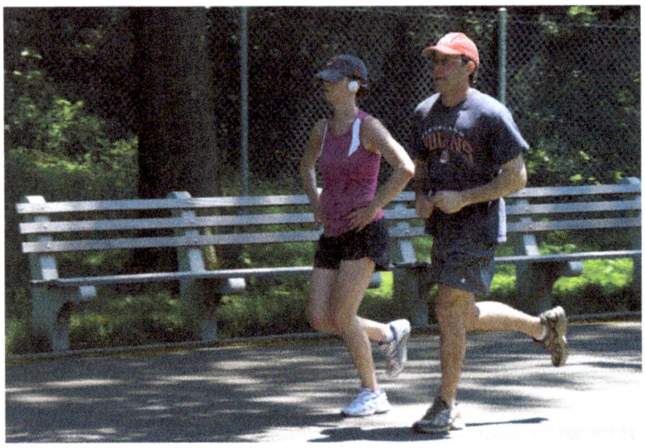

Jogging is one form of aerobic exercise.

Humans are genetically predisposed with a larger percentage of one type of muscle group over another. An individual born with a greater percentage of Type I muscle fibers would theoretically be more suited to endurance events, such as triathlons, distance running, and long cycling events, whereas a human born with a greater percentage of Type II muscle fibers would be more likely to excel at sprinting events such as 100 meter dash.

Exercise

Exercise is often recommended as a means of improving motor skills, fitness, muscle and bone strength, and joint function. Exercise has several effects upon muscles, connective tissue, bone, and the nerves that stimulate the muscles. One such effect is muscle hypertrophy, an increase in size. This is used in bodybuilding.

Various exercises require a predominance of certain muscle fiber utilization over another. Aerobic exercise involves long, low levels of exertion in which the muscles are used at well below their maximal contraction strength for long periods of time (the most classic example being the marathon). Aerobic events, which rely primarily on the aerobic (with oxygen) system, use a higher percentage of Type I (or slow-twitch) muscle fibers, consume a mixture of fat, protein and carbohydrates for energy, consume large amounts of oxygen and produce little lactic acid. Anaerobic exercise involves short bursts of higher intensity contractions at a much greater percentage of their maximum contraction strength. Examples of anaerobic exercise include sprinting and weight lifting. The anaerobic energy delivery system uses predominantly Type II or fast-twitch muscle fibers, relies mainly on ATP or glucose for fuel, consumes relatively little oxygen, protein and fat, produces large amounts of lactic acid and can not be sustained for as long a period as aerobic exercise. Many exercises are partially aerobic and partially anaerobic; for example, soccer and rock climbing involve a combination of both.

The presence of lactic acid has an inhibitory effect on ATP generation within the muscle; though not producing fatigue, it can inhibit or even stop performance if the intracellular concentration becomes too high. However, long-term training causes neovascularization within the muscle, increasing the ability to move waste products out of the muscles and maintain contraction. Once moved out of muscles with high concentrations within the sarcomere, lactic acid can be used by other muscles or body tissues as a source of energy, or transported to the liver where it is converted back to pyruvate. In addition to increasing the level of lactic acid, strenuous exercise causes the loss of potassium ions in muscle and causing an increase in potassium ion concentrations close to the muscle fibres, in the interstitium. Acidification by lactic acid may allow recovery of force so that acidosis may protect against fatigue rather than being a cause of fatigue.

Delayed onset muscle soreness is pain or discomfort that may be felt one to three days after exercising and generally subsides two to three days later. Once thought to be caused by lactic acid build-up, a more recent theory is that it is caused by tiny tears in the muscle fibers caused by eccentric contraction, or unaccustomed training levels. Since lactic acid disperses fairly rapidly, it could not explain pain experienced days after exercise.

Hypertrophy

Independent of strength and performance measures, muscles can be induced to grow larger by a number of factors, including hormone signaling, developmental factors, strength training, and disease. Contrary to popular belief, the number of muscle fibres cannot be increased through exercise. Instead, muscles grow larger through a combination of muscle cell growth as new protein filaments are added along with additional mass provided by undifferentiated satellite cells alongside the existing muscle cells.

Biological factors such as age and hormone levels can affect muscle hypertrophy. During puberty in males, hypertrophy occurs at an accelerated rate as the levels of growth-stimulating hormones produced by the body increase. Natural hypertrophy normally stops at full growth in the late teens. As testosterone is one of the body's major growth hormones, on average, men find hypertrophy much easier to achieve than women. Taking additional testosterone or other anabolic steroids will increase muscular hypertrophy.

Muscular, spinal and neural factors all affect muscle building. Sometimes a person may notice an increase in strength in a given muscle even though only its opposite has been subject to exercise, such as when a bodybuilder finds her left biceps stronger after completing a regimen focusing only on the right biceps. This phenomenon is called cross education.

Atrophy

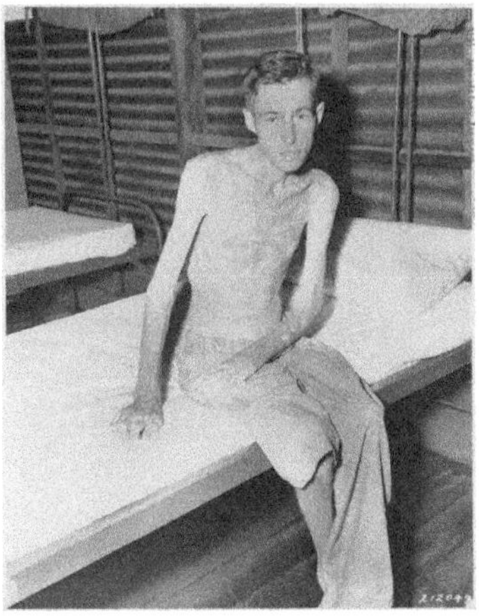

Prisoner of war exhibiting muscle loss as a result of malnutrition. Muscles may atrophy as a result of malnutrition, physical inactivity, aging, or disease.

Inactivity and starvation in mammals lead to atrophy of skeletal muscle, a decrease in muscle mass that may be accompanied by a smaller number and size of the muscle cells as well as lower protein content. Muscle atrophy may also result from the natural aging process or from disease.

In humans, prolonged periods of immobilization, as in the cases of bed rest or astronauts flying in space, are known to result in muscle weakening and atrophy. Atrophy is of particular interest to the manned spaceflight community, because the weightlessness experienced in spaceflight results is a loss of as much as 30% of mass in some muscles. Such consequences are also noted in small hibernating mammals like the golden-mantled ground squirrels and brown bats.

During aging, there is a gradual decrease in the ability to maintain skeletal muscle function and mass, known as sarcopenia. The exact cause of sarcopenia is unknown, but it may be due to a combination of the gradual failure in the "satellite cells" that help to regenerate skeletal muscle fibers, and a decrease in sensitivity to or the availability of critical secreted growth factors that are necessary to maintain muscle mass and satellite cell survival. Sarcopenia is a normal aspect of aging, and is not actually a disease state yet can be linked to many injuries in the elderly population as well as decreasing quality of life.

There are also many diseases and conditions that cause muscle atrophy. Examples include cancer and AIDS, which induce a body wasting syndrome called cachexia. Other syndromes or conditions that can induce skeletal muscle atrophy are congestive heart disease and some diseases of the liver.

Disease

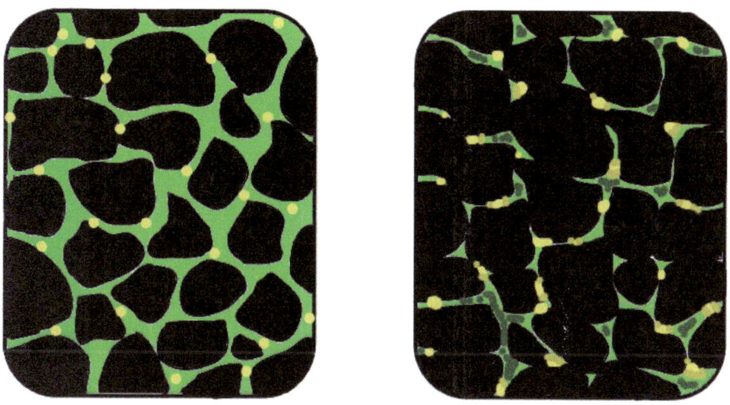

In muscular dystrophy, the affected tissues become disorganized and the concentration of dystrophin (green) is greatly reduced.

Neuromuscular diseases are those that affect the muscles and/or their nervous control. In general, problems with nervous control can cause spasticity or paralysis, depending on the location and nature of the problem. A large proportion of neurological disorders, ranging from cerebrovascular accident (stroke) and Parkinson's disease to Creutzfeldt–Jakob disease, can lead to problems with movement or motor coordination.

Symptoms of muscle diseases may include weakness, spasticity, myoclonus and myalgia. Diagnostic procedures that may reveal muscular disorders include testing creatine kinase levels in the blood and electromyography (measuring electrical activity in muscles). In some cases, muscle biopsy may be done to identify a myopathy, as well as genetic testing to identify DNA abnormalities associated with specific myopathies and dystrophies.

A non-invasive elastography technique that measures muscle noise is undergoing experimentation to provide a way of monitoring neuromuscular disease. The sound produced by a muscle comes from the shortening of actomyosin filaments along the axis of the muscle. During contraction, the muscle shortens along its longitudinal axis and expands across the transverse axis, producing vibrations at the surface.

Evolution

The evolutionary origin of muscle cells in metazoans is a highly debated topic. In one line of thought scientists have believed that muscle cells evolved once and thus all animals with muscles cells have a single common ancestor. In the other line of thought, scientists believe muscles cells evolved more than once and any morphological or structural similarities are due to convergent evolution and genes that predate the evolution of muscle and even the mesoderm - the germ layer from which many scientists believe true muscle cells derive.

Schmid and Seipel argue that the origin of muscle cells is a monophyletic trait that occurred concurrently with the development of the digestive and nervous systems of all animals and that this origin can be traced to a single metazoan ancestor in which muscle cells are present. They argue that molecular and morphological similarities between the muscles cells in cnidaria and ctenophora are similar enough to those of bilaterians that there would be one ancestor in metazoans from which muscle cells derive. In this case, Schmid and Seipel argue that the last common ancestor of bilateria, ctenophora, and cnidaria was a triploblast or an organism with three germ layers and that diploblasty, meaning an organism with two germ layers, evolved secondarily due to their observation of the lack of mesoderm or muscle found in most cnidarians and ctenophores. By comparing the morphology of cnidarians and ctenophores to bilaterians, Schmid and Seipel were able to conclude that there were myoblast-like structures in the tentacles and gut of some species of cnidarians and in the tentacles of ctenophores. Since this is a structure unique to muscle cells, these scientists determined based on the data collected by their peers that this is a marker for striated muscles similar to that observed in bilaterians. The authors also remark that the muscle cells found in cnidarians and ctenophores are often contests due to the origin of these muscle cells being the ectoderm rather than the mesoderm or mesendoderm. The origin of true muscles cells is argued by others to be the endoderm portion of the mesoderm and the endoderm. However, Schmid and Seipel counter this skepticism about whether or not the muscle cells found in ctenophores and cnidarians are true muscle cells by considering that cnidarians develop through a medusa stage and polyp stage. They observe that in the hydrozoan medusa stage there is a layer of cells that separate from the distal side of the ectoderm to form the striated muscle cells in a way that seems similar to that of the mesoderm and call this third separated layer of cells the ectocodon. They also argue that not all muscle cells are derived from the mesendoderm in bilaterians with key examples being that in both the eye muscles of vertebrates and the muscles of spiralians these cells derive from the ectodermal mesoderm rather than the endodermal mesoderm. Furthermore, Schmid and Seipel argue that since myogenesis does occur in cnidarians with the help of molecular regulatory elements found in the specification of muscles cells in bilaterians that there is evidence for a single origin for striated muscle.

In contrast to this argument for a single origin of muscle cells, Steinmetz et al. argue that molecular markers such as the myosin II protein used to determine this single origin of striated muscle actually predate the formation of muscle cells. This author uses an example of the contractile elements present in the porifera or sponges that do truly lack this striated muscle containing this protein. Furthermore, Steinmetz et al. present evidence for a polyphyletic origin of striated muscle cell development through their analysis of morphological and molecular markers that are present in bilaterians and absent in cnidarians, ctenophores, and bilaterians. Steimetz et al. showed that the traditional morphological and regulatory markers such as actin, the ability to couple myosin side chains phosphorylation to higher concentrations of the positive concentrations of calcium, and other MyHC elements are present in all metazoans not just the organisms that have been shown to have muscle cells. Thus, the usage of any of these structural or regulatory elements in determining whether or not the muscle cells of the cnidarians and ctenophores are similar enough to the muscle cells of the bilaterians to confirm a single lineage is questionable according to Steinmetz et al. Furthermore, Steinmetz et al. explain that the orthologues of the MyHc genes that have been used to hypothesize the origin of striated muscle occurred through a gene duplication event that predates the first true muscle cells (meaning striated muscle), and they show that the MyHc genes are present in the sponges that have contractile elements but no true muscle cells. Furthermore, Steinmetz et all showed that the localization of this duplicated set of genes that serve both the function of facilitating the formation of striated muscle genes and cell regulation and movement genes were already separated into striated myhc and non-muscle myhc. This separation of the duplicated set of genes is shown through the localization of the striated myhc to the contractile vacuole in sponges while the non-muscle myhc was more diffusely expressed during developmental cell shape and change. Steinmetz et al. found a similar pattern of localization in cnidarians with except with the cnidarian *N. vectensis* having this striated muscle marker present in the smooth muscle of the digestive track. Thus, Steinmetz et al. argue that the pleisiomorphic trait of the separated orthologues of myhc cannot be used to determine the monophylogeny of muscle, and additionally argue that the presence of a striated muscle marker in the smooth muscle of this cnidarian shows a fundamentally different mechanism of muscle cell development and structure in cnidarians.

Steinmetz et al. continue to argue for multiple origins of striated muscle in the metazoans by explaining that a key set of genes used to form the troponin complex for muscle regulation and formation in bilaterians is missing from the cnidarians and ctenophores, and of 47 structural and regulatory proteins observed, Steinmetz et al. were not able to find even on unique striated muscle cell protein that was expressed in both cnidarians and bilaterians. Furthermore, the Z-disc seemed to have evolved differently even within bilaterians and there is a great deal diversity of proteins developed even between this clade, showing a large degree of radiation for muscle cells. Through this divergence of the Z-disc, Steimetz et al. argue that there are only four common protein components that were present in all bilaterians muscle ancestors and that of these for necessary Z-disc components only an actin protein that they have already argued is an uninformative marker through its pleisiomorphic state is present in cnidarians. Through further molecular marker testing, Steinmetz et al. observe that non-bilaterians lack many regulatory and structural components necessary for bilaterians muscle formation and do not find any unique set of proteins to both bilaterians and cnidarians and ctenophores that are not present in earlier, more primitive animals such as the sponges and amoebozoans. Through this analysis the authors conclude that due to the lack of elements that bilaterians muscles are dependent on for structure and usage, nonbilaterian muscles must be of a different origin with a different set regulatory and structural proteins.

In another take on the argument, Andrikou and Arnone use the newly available data on gene regulatory networks to look at how the hierarchy of genes and morphogens and other mechanism of tissue specification diverge and are similar among early deuterostomes and protostomes. By understanding not only what genes are present in all bilaterians but also the time and place of deployment of these genes, Andrikou and Arnone discuss a deeper understanding of the evolution of myogenesis.

In their paper Andrikou and Arnone argue that to truly understand the evolution of muscle cells the function of transcriptional regulators must be understood in the context of other external and internal interactions. Through their analysis, Andrikou and Arnone found that there were conserved orthologues of the gene regulatory network in both invertebrate bilaterians and in cnidarians. They argue that having this common, general regulatory circuit allowed for a high degree of divergence from a single well functioning network. Andrikou and Arnone found that the orthologues of genes found in vertebrates had been changed through different types of structural mutations in the invertebrate deuterostomes and protostomes, and they argue that these structural changes in the genes allowed for a large divergence of muscle function and muscle formation in these species. Andrikou and Arnone were able to recognize not only any difference due to mutation in the genes found in vertebrates and invertebrates but also the integration of species specific genes that could also cause divergence from the original gene regulatory network function. Thus, although a common muscle patterning system has been determined, they argue that this could be due to a more ancestral gene regulatory network being coopted several times across lineages with additional genes and mutations causing very divergent development of muscles. Thus it seems that myogenic patterning framework may be an ancestral trait. However, Andrikou and Arnone explain that the basic muscle patterning structure must also be considered in combination with the cis regulatory elements present at different times during development. In contrast with the high level of gene family apparatuses structure, Andrikou and Arnone found that the cis regulatory elements were not well conserved both in time and place in the network which could show a large degree of divergence in the formation of muscle cells. Through this analysis, it seems that the myogenic GRN is an ancestral GRN with actual changes in myogenic function and structure possibly being linked to later coopts of genes at different times and places.

Evolutionarily, specialized forms of skeletal and cardiac muscles predated the divergence of the vertebrate/arthropod evolutionary line. This indicates that these types of muscle developed in a common ancestor sometime before 700 million years ago (mya). Vertebrate smooth muscle was found to have evolved independently from the skeletal and cardiac muscle types.

Skeletal Muscle

Skeletal muscle is one of three major muscle types, the others being cardiac muscle and smooth muscle. It is a form of striated muscle tissue which is under the 'voluntary' control of the somatic nervous system. Most skeletal muscles are attached to bones by bundles of collagen fibers known as tendons.

A skeletal muscle refers to multiple bundles of cells called muscle fibers (fascicles). The fibres and muscles are surrounded by connective tissue layers called fasciae. Muscle fibres, or muscle cells, are formed from the fusion of developmental myoblasts in a process known as myogenesis. Muscle fibres are cylindrical, and have more than one nucleus.

Muscle fibers are in turn composed of myofibrils. The myofibrils are composed of actin and myosin filaments, repeated in units called sarcomeres, which are the basic functional units of the muscle fiber. The sarcomere is responsible for the striated appearance of skeletal muscle, and forms the basic machinery necessary for muscle contraction.

Skeletal Muscles

Connective tissue is present in all muscles as fascia. Enclosing each muscle is a layer of connective tissue known as the epimysium; enclosing each fascicle is a layer called the perimysium, and enclosing each muscle fiber is a layer of connective tissue called the endomysium.

Muscle Fibers

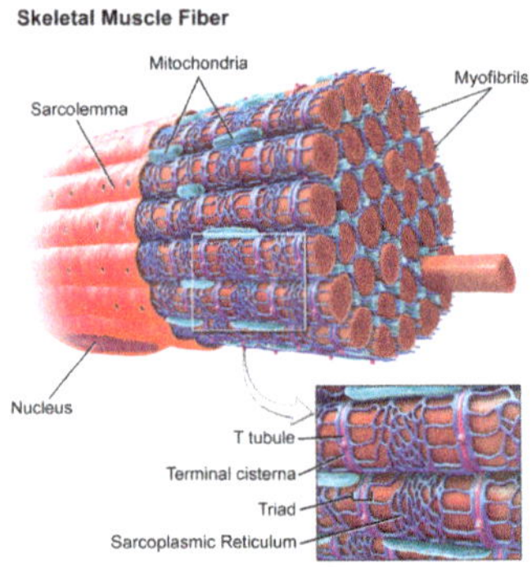

Skeletal muscle fiber

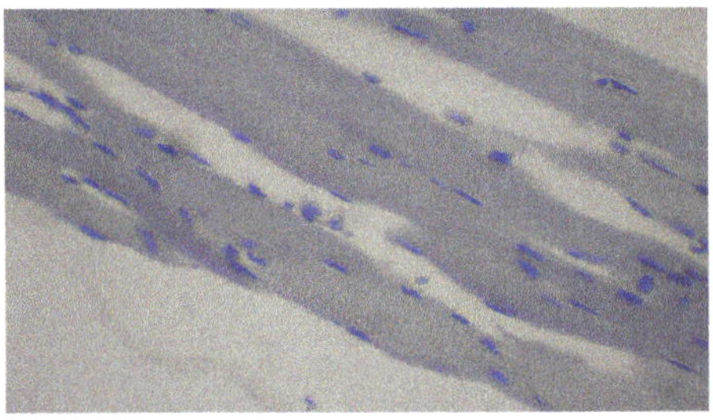

Skeletal muscle fibers show sarcomeres clearly

Muscle fibres are the individual contractile units within muscle. A single muscle such as the biceps brachii contains many muscle fibres.

Another group of cells, the myosatellite cells are found between the basement membrane and the sarcolemma of muscle fibers. These cells are normally quiescent but can be activated by exercise or pathology to provide additional myonuclei for muscle growth or repair.

Development

Individual muscle fibers are formed during development from the fusion of several undifferentiated immature cells known as myoblasts into long, cylindrical, multi-nucleated cells. Differentiation into this state is primarily completed before birth with the cells continuing to grow in size thereafter.

Microanatomy

Skeletal muscle exhibits a distinctive banding pattern when viewed under the microscope due to the arrangement of cytoskeletal elements in the cytoplasm of the muscle fibers. The principal cytoplasmic proteins are myosin and actin (also known as "thick" and "thin" filaments, respectively) which are arranged in a repeating unit called a sarcomere. The interaction of myosin and actin is responsible for muscle contraction.

Every single organelle and macromolecule of a muscle fiber is arranged to ensure form meets function. The cell membrane is called the sarcolemma with the cytoplasm known as the sarcoplasm. In the sarcoplasm are the myofibrils. The myofibrils are long protein bundles about 1 micrometer in diameter each containing myofilaments. Pressed against the inside of the sarcolemma are the unusual flattened myonuclei. Between the myofibrils are the mitochondria.

While the muscle fiber does not have a smooth endoplasmic reticulum, it contains a sarcoplasmic reticulum. The sarcoplasmic reticulum surrounds the myofibrils and holds a reserve of the calcium ions needed to cause a muscle contraction. Periodically, it has dilated end sacs known as terminal cisternae. These cross the muscle fiber from one side to the other. In between two terminal cisternae is a tubular infolding called a transverse tubule (T tubule). T tubules are the pathways for action potentials to signal the sarcoplasmic reticulum to release calcium, causing a muscle contraction. Together, two terminal cisternae and a transverse tubule form a triad.

Arrangement of Muscle Fibres

Muscle architecture refers to the arrangement of muscle fibers relative to the axis of force generation of the muscle. This axis is a hypothetical line from the muscle's origin to insertion. For some longitudinal muscles, such as the biceps brachii, this is a relatively simple concept. For others, such as the rectus femoris or deltoid muscle, it becomes more complicated. While the muscle fibers of a fascicle lie parallel to one another, the fascicles themselves can vary in their relationship to one another and to their tendons. The different fiber arrangements produce broad categories of skeletal muscle architectures including longitudinal, pennate, unipennate, bipennate, and multipennate. Because of these different architectures, the tension a muscle can create between its tendons varies by more than simply its size and fiber-type makeup.

Longitudinal Architecture

The fascicles of longitudinally arranged, parallel, or fusiform muscles run parallel to the axis of force generation, thus these muscles on a whole function similarly to a single, large muscle fiber. Variations exist, and the different terms are often used more specifically. For instance, fusiform refers to a longitudinal architecture with a widened muscle belly (biceps), while parallel may refer to a more ribon-shaped longitudinal architecture (rectus abdominis). A less common example would be a circular muscle such as the orbicularis oris, in which the fibers are longitudinally arranged, but create a circle from origin to insertion.

Unipennate Architecture

The fibers in unipennate muscles are all oriented at the same (but non-zero) angle relative to the axis of force generation. This angle reduces the effective force of any individual fiber, as it is effectively pulling off-axis. However, because of this angle, more fibers can be packed into the same muscle volume, increasing the Physiological cross-sectional area (PCSA). This effect is known as fiber packing, and—in terms of force generation—it more than overcomes the efficiency loss of the off-axis orientation. The trade-off comes in overall speed of muscle shortening and in total excursion. Overall muscle shortening speed is reduced compared to fiber shortening speed, as is the total distance of shortening. All of these effects scale with pennation angle; greater angles lead to greater force due to increased fiber packing and PCSA, but with greater losses in shortening speed and excursion. The vastus lateralis is an example of unipennate architecture.

Multipennate Architectures

The fibers in multipennate muscles are arranged at multiple angles in relation to the axis of force generation, and are the most general and most common architecture. Several fiber orientations fall into this category; bipennate, convergent, and multipennate. While the determination of PCSA becomes more difficult in these muscle architectures, the same tradeoffs apply.

Bipennate arrangements are essentially "V"s of fibers stacked on top of each other, such as in the rectus femoris.

Convergent arrangements are triangle or fan shaped, with wide origins and more narrow insertions. The wide variation of pennation angles in this architecture can actually allow for multiple functions. For instance, the trapezius, a prototypical convergent muscle, can aid in both shoulder elevation and depression.

Multipennate arrangements are not limited to a particular arrangement, but—when used specifically—commonly refer to what is essentially a combination of bipennate or unipennate arrangements with convergent arrangements. An example of this architecture would be the human deltoid muscle.

Function

Cellular Physiology and Contraction

In addition to the actin and myosin components that constitute the sarcomere, skeletal muscle fibers also contain two other important regulatory proteins, troponin and tropomyosin, that are necessary for muscle contraction to occur. These proteins are associated with actin and cooperate to prevent its interaction with myosin. Skeletal muscle cells are excitable and are subject to depolarization by the neurotransmitter acetylcholine, released at the neuromuscular junction by motor neurons.

Once a cell is sufficiently stimulated, the cell's sarcoplasmic reticulum releases ionic calcium (Ca2+), which then interacts with the regulatory protein troponin. Calcium-bound troponin undergoes a conformational change that leads to the movement of tropomyosin, subsequently exposing the myosin-binding sites on actin. This allows for myosin and actin ATP-dependent cross-bridge cycling and shortening of the muscle.

Physics

Muscle force is proportional to physiologic cross-sectional area (PCSA), and muscle velocity is proportional to muscle fiber length. The torque around a joint, however, is determined by a number of biomechanical parameters, including the distance between muscle insertions and pivot points, muscle size and Architectural gear ratio. Muscles are normally arranged in opposition so that when one group of muscles contracts, another group relaxes or lengthens. Antagonism in the transmission of nerve impulses to the muscles means that it is impossible to fully stimulate the contraction of two antagonistic muscles at any one time. During ballistic motions such as throwing, the antagonist muscles act to 'brake' the agonist muscles throughout the contraction, particularly at the end of the motion. In the example of throwing, the chest and front of the shoulder (anterior Deltoid) contract to pull the arm forward, while the muscles in the back and rear of the shoulder (posterior Deltoid) also contract and undergo eccentric contraction to slow the motion down to avoid injury. Part of the training process is learning to relax the antagonist muscles to increase the force input of the chest and anterior shoulder.

Contracting muscles produce vibration and sound. Slow twitch fibers produce 10 to 30 contractions per second (10 to 30 Hz). Fast twitch fibers produce 30 to 70 contractions per second (30 to 70 Hz). The vibration can be witnessed and felt by highly tensing one's muscles, as when making a firm fist. The sound can be heard by pressing a highly tensed muscle against the ear, again a firm fist is a good example. The sound is usually described as a rumbling sound. Some individuals can voluntarily produce this rumbling sound by contracting the tensor tympani muscle of the middle ear. The rumbling sound can also be heard when the neck or jaw muscles are highly tensed.

Signal Transduction Pathways

Skeletal muscle fiber-type phenotype in adult animals is regulated by several independent signaling pathways. These include pathways involved with the Ras/mitogen-activated protein kinase (MAPK) pathway, calcineurin, calcium/calmodulin-dependent protein kinase IV, and the peroxisome proliferator γ coactivator 1 (PGC-1). The Ras/MAPK signaling pathway links the motor neurons and signaling systems, coupling excitation and transcription regulation to promote the nerve-dependent induction of the slow program in regenerating muscle. Calcineurin, a Ca2+/calmodulin-activated phosphatase implicated in nerve activity-dependent fiber-type specification in skeletal muscle, directly controls the phosphorylation state of the transcription factor NFAT, allowing for its translocation to the nucleus and leading to the activation of slow-type muscle proteins in cooperation with myocyte enhancer factor 2 (MEF2) proteins and other regulatory proteins. Ca2+/calmodulin-dependent protein kinase activity is also upregulated by slow motor neuron activity, possibly because it amplifies the slow-type calcineurin-generated responses by promoting MEF2 transactivator functions and enhancing oxidative capacity through stimulation of mitochondrial biogenesis.

Contraction-induced changes in intracellular calcium or reactive oxygen species provide signals to diverse pathways that include the MAPKs, calcineurin and calcium/calmodulin-dependent protein kinase IV to activate transcription factors that regulate gene expression and enzyme activity in skeletal muscle.

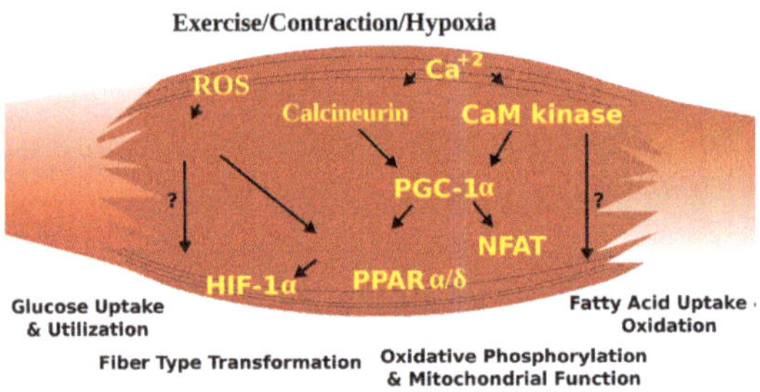

Exercise-Included Signaling Pathways in Skeletal Muscle That Determine Specialized Characteristics of slow twitch and fast twitch Muscle Fibers.

PGC1-α (PPARGC1A), a transcriptional coactivator of nuclear receptors important to the regulation of a number of mitochondrial genes involved in oxidative metabolism, directly interacts with MEF2 to synergistically activate selective slow twitch (ST) muscle genes and also serves as a target for calcineurin signaling. A peroxisome proliferator-activated receptor δ (PPARδ)-mediated transcriptional pathway is involved in the regulation of the skeletal muscle fiber phenotype. Mice that harbor an activated form of PPARd display an "endurance" phenotype, with a coordinated increase in oxidative enzymes and mitochondrial biogenesis and an increased proportion of ST fibers. Thus—through functional genomics—calcineurin, calmodulin-dependent kinase, PGC-1α, and activated PPARδ form the basis of a signaling network that controls skeletal muscle fiber-type transformation and metabolic profiles that protect against insulin resistance and obesity.

The transition from aerobic to anaerobic metabolism during intense work requires that several systems are rapidly activated to ensure a constant supply of ATP for the working muscles. These include a switch from fat-based to carbohydrate-based fuels, a redistribution of blood flow from nonworking to exercising muscles, and the removal of several of the by-products of anaerobic metabolism, such as carbon dioxide and lactic acid. Some of these responses are governed by transcriptional control of the fast twtich (FT) glycolytic phenotype. For example, skeletal muscle reprogramming from an ST glycolytic phenotype to an FT glycolytic phenotype involves the Six1/Eya1 complex, composed of members of the Six protein family. Moreover, the hypoxia-inducible factor 1-α (HIF1A) has been identified as a master regulator for the expression of genes involved in essential hypoxic responses that maintain ATP levels in cells. Ablation of HIF-1α in skeletal muscle was associated with an increase in the activity of rate-limiting enzymes of the mitochondria, indicating that the citric acid cycle and increased fatty acid oxidation may be compensating for decreased flow through the glycolytic pathway in these animals. However, hypoxia-mediated HIF-1α responses are also linked to the regulation of mitochondrial dysfunction through the formation of excessive reactive oxygen species in mitochondria.

Other pathways also influence adult muscle character. For example, physical force inside a muscle fiber may release the transcription factor serum response factor (SRF) from the structural protein titin, leading to altered muscle growth.

Clinical Significance

Diseases of skeletal muscle are termed Myopathies, while diseases of nerves are called Neuropathies. Both can affect muscle function and/or cause muscle pain, and fall under the umbrella of Neuromuscular disease. Myopathies have been modeled with cell culture systems of muscle from healthy or diseased tissue biopsies. Another source of skeletal muscle and progenitors is provided by the directed differentiation of pluripotent stem cells .

Research

Research on skeletal muscle properties uses many techniques. Electrical muscle stimulation is used to determine force and contraction speed at different stimulation frequencies, which are related to fiber-type composition and mix within an individual muscle group. In vitro muscle testing is used for more complete characterization of muscle properties.

The electrical activity associated with muscle contraction are measured via electromyography (EMG). EMG is a common technique used in many disciplines within the Exercise and Rehab Sciences. Skeletal muscle has two physiological responses: relaxation and contraction. The mechanisms for which these responses occur generate electrical activity measured by EMG. Specifically, EMG can measure the action potential of a skeletal muscle, which occurs from the hyperpolarization of the motor axons from nerve impulses sent to the muscle (1). EMG is used in research for determining if the skeletal muscle of interest is being activated, the amount of force generated, and an indicator of muscle fatigue. The two types of EMG are intra-muscular EMG and the most common, surface EMG. The EMG signals are much greater when a skeletal muscle is contracting verses relaxing. However, for smaller and deeper skeletal muscles the EMG signals are reduced and therefore are viewed as a less valued technique for measuring the activation. In research using EMG, a maximal voluntary contraction (MVC) is commonly performed on the skeletal muscle of interest, to have reference data for the rest of the EMG recordings during the main experimental testing for that same skeletal muscle.

B. K. Pedersen and her colleagues have conducted research showing that skeletal muscle functions as an endocrine organ by secreting cytokines and other peptides, now referred to as myokines. Myokines in turn are believed to mediate the health benefits of exercise.

Cardiac Muscle

Cardiac muscle (heart muscle) is an involuntary, striated muscle that is found in the walls and histological foundation of the heart, specifically the myocardium. Cardiac muscle is one of three major types of muscle, the others being skeletal and smooth muscle. These three types of muscle all form in the process of myogenesis. The cells that constitute cardiac muscle, called cardiomyocytes or myocardiocytes, predominantly contain only one nucleus, although populations with two to four nuclei do exist. The myocardium is the muscle tissue of the heart, and forms a thick middle layer between the outer epicardium layer and the inner endocardium layer.

Coordinated contractions of cardiac muscle cells in the heart pump blood out of the atria and ventricles to the blood vessels of the left/body/systemic and right/lungs/pulmonary circulatory systems. This complex mechanism illustrates systole of the heart.

Cardiac muscle cells, unlike most other tissues in the body, rely on an available blood and electrical supply to deliver oxygen and nutrients and remove waste products such as carbon dioxide. The coronary arteries help fulfill this function.

Structure

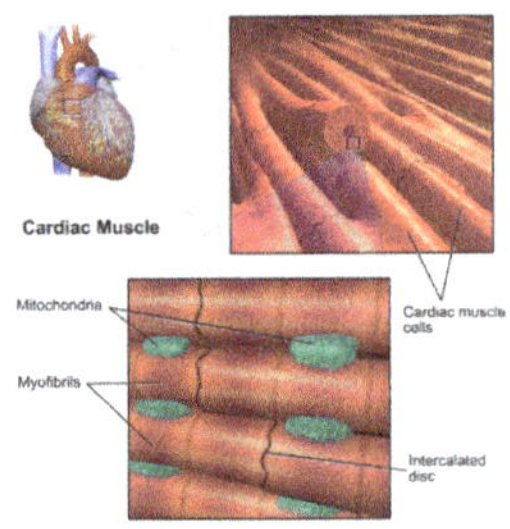

Cardiac muscle

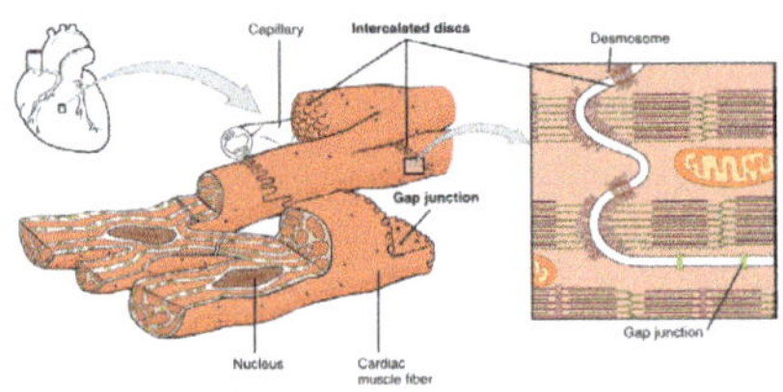

Intercalated discs are part of the cardiac muscle sarcolemma and they contain gap junctions and desmosomes.

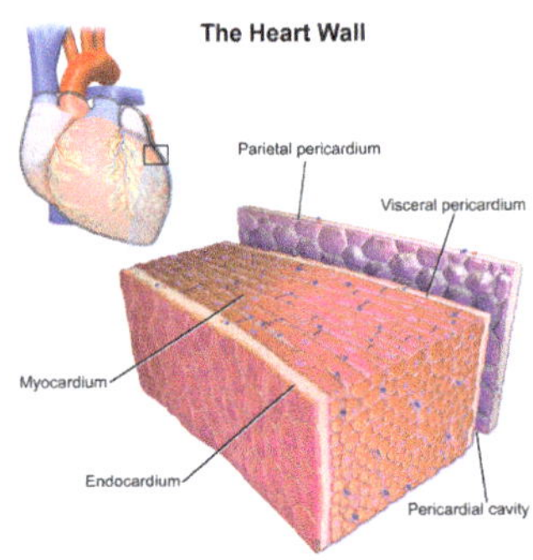

Thick myocardium within heart wall.

Striation

Cardiac muscle has cross striations formed by rotating segments of thick and thin protein filaments. Like skeletal muscle, the primary structural proteins of cardiac muscle are myosin and actin. The actin filaments are thin, causing the lighter appearance of the I bands in striated muscle, whereas the myosin filament is thicker, lending a darker appearance to the alternating A bands as observed with electron microscopy. However, in contrast to skeletal muscle, cardiac muscle cells are typically branch-like instead of linear.

T-tubules

Another histological difference between cardiac muscle and skeletal muscle is that the T-tubules in the cardiac muscle are bigger and wider and track laterally to the Z-discs. There are fewer T-tubules in comparison with skeletal muscle. The diad is a structure in the cardiac myocyte located at the sarcomere Z-line. It is composed of a single T-tubule paired with a terminal cisterna of the sarcoplasmic reticulum. The diad plays an important role in excitation-contraction coupling by juxtaposing an inlet for the action potential near a source of Ca^{2+} ions. This way, the wave of depolarization can be coupled to calcium-mediated cardiac muscle contraction via the sliding filament mechanism. Cardiac muscle forms these instead of the triads formed between the sarcoplasmic reticulum in skeletal muscle and T-tubules. T-tubules play critical role in excitation-contraction coupling (ECC). Recently, the action potentials of T-tubules were recorded optically by Guixue Bu et al.

Intercalated Discs

The cardiac syncytium is a network of cardiomyocytes connected to each other by intercalated discs that enable the rapid transmission of electrical impulses through the network, enabling the syncytium to act in a coordinated contraction of the myocardium. There is an atrial syncytium and a ventricular syncytium that are connected by cardiac connection fibres. Electrical resistance through intercalated discs is very low, thus allowing free diffusion of ions. The ease of ion movement along cardiac muscle fibers axes is such that action potentials are able to travel from one cardiac muscle cell to the next, facing only slight resistance. Each syncytium obeys the all or none law.

Intercalated discs are complex adhering structures that connect the single cardiomyocytes to an electrochemical syncytium (in contrast to the skeletal muscle, which becomes a multicellular syncytium during mammalian embryonic development). The discs are responsible mainly for force transmission during muscle contraction. Intercalated discs consist of three different types of cell-cell junctions: the actin filament anchoring adherens junctions, the intermediate filament anchoring desmosomes , and gap junctions. They allow action potentials to spread between cardiac cells by permitting the passage of ions between cells, producing depolarization of the heart muscle.

However, novel molecular biological and comprehensive studies unequivocally showed that intercalated discs consist for the most part of mixed-type adhering junctions named *area composita* (pl. *areae compositae*) representing an amalgamation of typical desmosomal and *fascia adhaerens* proteins (in contrast to various epithelia). The authors discuss the high importance of these findings for the understanding of inherited cardiomyopathies (such as arrhythmogenic right ventricular cardiomyopathy).

Under light microscopy, intercalated discs appear as thin, typically dark-staining lines dividing adjacent cardiac muscle cells. The intercalated discs run perpendicular to the direction of muscle fibers. Under electron microscopy, an intercalated disc's path appears more complex. At low magnification, this may appear as a convoluted electron dense structure overlying the location of the obscured Z-line. At high magnification, the intercalated disc's path appears even more convoluted, with both longitudinal and transverse areas appearing in longitudinal section.

Physiology

In contrast to skeletal muscle, cardiac muscle requires *extracellular calcium ions* for contraction to occur. Like skeletal muscle, the initiation and upshoot of the action potential in ventricular cardiomyocytes is derived from the entry of sodium ions across the sarcolemma in a regenerative process. However, an inward flux of extracellular calcium ions through L-type calcium channels sustains the depolarization of cardiac muscle cells for a longer duration. The reason for the calcium dependence is due to the mechanism of calcium-induced calcium release (CICR) from the sarcoplasmic reticulum that must occur during normal excitation-contraction (EC) coupling to cause contraction. Once the intracellular concentration of calcium increases, calcium ions bind to the protein troponin, which allows myosin to bind to actin and contraction to occur.

Regeneration of Heart Muscle Cells

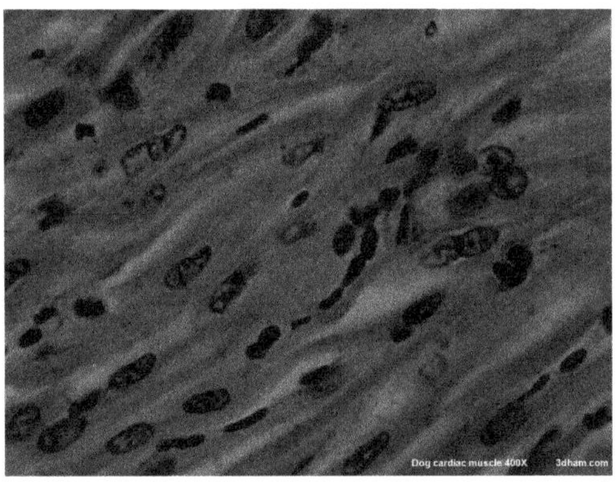

Dog cardiac muscle (400X)

Until recently, it was commonly believed that cardiac muscle cells could not be regenerated. However, a study reported in the April 3, 2009 issue of *Science* contradicts that belief. Olaf Bergmann and his colleagues at the Karolinska Institute in Stockholm tested samples of heart muscle from people born before 1955 who had very little cardiac muscle around their heart, many showing with disabilities from this abnormality. By using DNA samples from many hearts, the researchers estimated that a 4-year-old renews about 20% of heart muscle cells per year, and about 69 percent of the heart muscle cells of a 50-year-old were generated after he or she was born.

One way that cardiomyocyte regeneration occurs is through the division of pre-existing cardiomyocytes during the normal aging process. The division process of pre-existing cardiomyocytes has also been shown to increase in areas adjacent to sites of myocardial injury. In addition, certain growth factors promote the self-renewal of endogenous cardiomyocytes and cardiac stem cells. For example, insulin-like growth factor 1, hepatocyte growth factor, and high-mobility group protein B1 increase cardiac stem cell migration to the affected area, as well as the proliferation and survival of these cells. Some members of the fibroblast growth factor family also induce cell-cycle re-entry of small cardiomyocytes. Vascular endothelial growth factor also plays an important role in the recruitment of native cardiac cells to an infarct site in addition to its angiogenic effect.

Based on the natural role of stem cells in cardiomyocyte regeneration, researchers and clinicians are increasingly interested in using these cells to induce regeneration of damaged tissue. Various stem cell lineages have been shown to be able to differentiate into cardiomyocytes, including bone marrow stem cells. For example, in one study, researchers transplanted bone marrow cells, which included a population of stem cells, adjacent to an infarct site in a mouse model. Nine days after surgery, the researchers found a new band of regenerating myocardium. However, this regeneration was not observed when the injected population of cells was devoid of stem cells, which strongly suggests that it was the stem cell population that contributed to the myocardium regeneration. Other clinical trials have shown that autologous bone marrow cell transplants delivered via the infarct-related artery decreases the infarct area compared to patients not given the cell therapy.

Clinical Significance

Occlusion (blockage) of the coronary arteries by atherosclerosis and/or thrombosis can lead to myocardial infarction (heart attack), where part of the myocardium is injured due to ischemia (not receiving enough oxygen). This occurs because coronary arteries are functional end arteries - i.e. there is almost no overlap in the areas supplied by different arteries (anastomoses) so that if one fails, others cannot adequately perfuse the region, unlike in other tissues.

Certain viruses lead to myocarditis (inflammation of the myocardium). Cardiomyopathies are inherent diseases of the myocardium, many of which are caused by genetic mutations.

Muscle Contraction

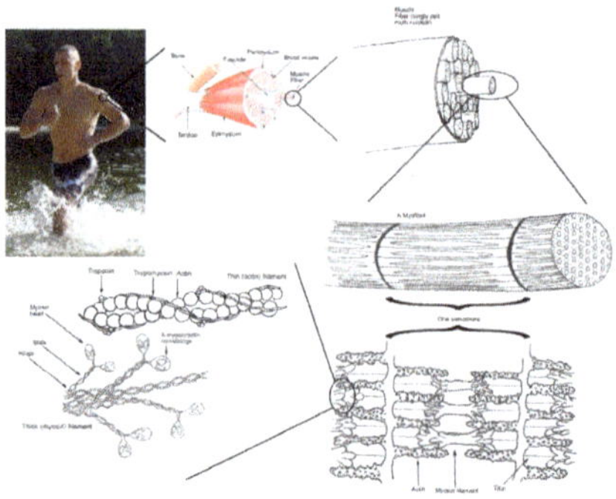

Hierarchical organization of skeletal muscle

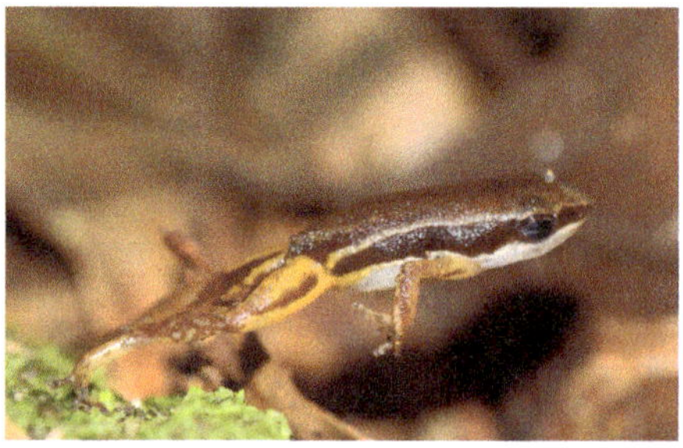

Contractions of skeletal muscles allow vertebrate animals such as frogs to move

Muscle contraction is the activation of tension-generating sites within muscle fibers. In physiology, muscle contraction does not necessarily mean muscle shortening because muscle tension can be produced without changes in muscle length such as holding a heavy book or a dumbbell at the same position. The termination of muscle contraction is followed by muscle relaxation, which is a return of the muscle fibers to their low tension-generating state.

Muscle contractions can be described based on two variables: length and tension. A muscle contraction is described as isometric if the muscle tension changes but the muscle length remains the same. In contrast, a muscle contraction is isotonic if muscle length changes but the muscle tension remains the same. If the muscle length shortens, the contraction is concentric; if the muscle length lengthens, the contraction is eccentric. In natural movements that underlie locomotor activity, muscle contractions are multifaceted as they are able to produce changes in length and tension in a time-varying manner. Therefore, neither length nor tension is likely to remain the same in muscles that contract during locomotor activity.

In vertebrates, skeletal muscle contractions are neurogenic as they require synaptic input from motor neurons to produce muscle contractions. A single motor neuron is able to innervate multiple muscle fibers, thereby causing the fibers to contract at the same time. Once innervated, the protein filaments within each skeletal muscle fiber slide past each other to produce a contraction, which is explained by the sliding filament theory. The contraction produced can be described as a twitch, summation, or tetanus, depending on the frequency of action potentials. In skeletal muscles, muscle tension is at its greatest when the muscle is stretched to an intermediate length as described by the length-tension relationship.

Unlike skeletal muscle, the contractions of smooth and cardiac muscles are myogenic (meaning that they are initiated by the smooth or heart muscle cells themselves instead of being stimulated by an outside event such as nerve stimulation), although they can be modulated by stimuli from the autonomic nervous system. The mechanisms of contraction in these muscle tissues are similar to those in skeletal muscle tissues.

Types

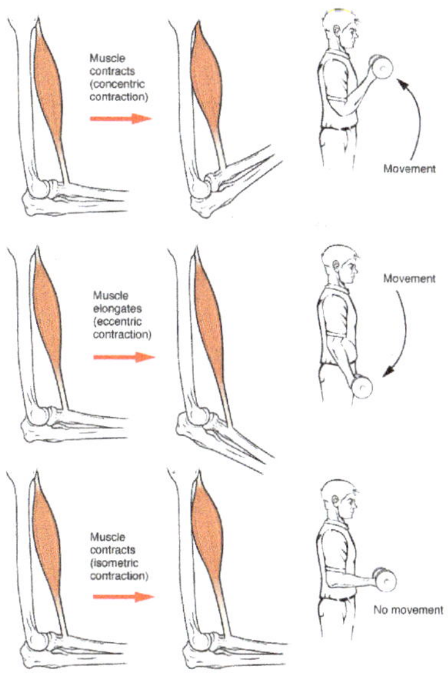

Types of muscle contractions

Muscle contractions can be described based on two variables: force and length. Force itself can be differentiated as either tension or load. Muscle tension is the force exerted by the muscle on an object whereas a load is the force exerted by an object on the muscle. When muscle tension changes without any corresponding changes in muscle length, the muscle contraction is described as isometric. If the muscle length changes while muscle tension remains the same, then the muscle contraction is isotonic. In an isotonic contraction, the muscle length can either shorten to produce a concentric contraction or lengthen to produce an eccentric contraction. Furthermore, if the muscle length shortens, the contraction is concentric. But if the muscle length lengthens, then the contraction is eccentric. In natural movements that underlie locomotor activity, muscle contractions are multifaceted as they are able to produce changes in length and tension in a time-varying manner. Therefore, neither length nor tension is likely to remain constant when the muscle is active during locomotor activity.

Isometric Contraction

An isometric contraction of a muscle generates tension without changing length. An example can be found when the muscles of the hand and forearm grip an object; the joints of the hand do not move, but muscles generate sufficient force to prevent the object from being dropped.

Isotonic Contraction

In isotonic contraction, the tension in the muscle remains constant despite a change in muscle length. This occurs when a muscle's force of contraction matches the total load on the muscle.

Concentric Contraction

In concentric contraction, muscle tension is sufficient to overcome the load, and the muscle shortens as it contracts. This occurs when the force generated by the muscle exceeds the load opposing its contraction.

During a concentric contraction, a muscle is stimulated to contract according to the sliding filament theory. This occurs throughout the length of the muscle, generating a force at the origin and insertion, causing the muscle to shorten and changing the angle of the joint. In relation to the elbow, a concentric contraction of the biceps would cause the arm to bend at the elbow as the hand moved from the leg to the shoulder (a biceps curl). A concentric contraction of the triceps would change the angle of the joint in the opposite direction, straightening the arm and moving the hand towards the leg.

Eccentric Contraction

In *eccentric contraction*, the tension generated is insufficient to overcome the external load on the muscle and the muscle fibers lengthen as they contract. Rather than working to pull a joint in the direction of the muscle contraction, the muscle acts to decelerate the joint at the end of a movement or otherwise control the repositioning of a load. This can occur involuntarily (e.g., when attempting to move a weight too heavy for the muscle to lift) or voluntarily (e.g., when the muscle is 'smoothing out' a movement). Over the short-term, strength training involving both eccentric and concentric contractions appear to increase muscular strength more than training with concentric contractions alone. However, exercise-induced muscle damage is also greater during lengthening contractions.

During an eccentric contraction of the biceps muscle, the elbow starts the movement while bent and then straightens as the hand moves away from the shoulder. During an eccentric contraction of the triceps muscle, the elbow starts the movement straight and then bends as the hand moves towards the shoulder. Desmin, titin, and other z-line proteins are involved in eccentric contractions, but their mechanism is poorly understood in comparison to crossbridge cycling in concentric contractions.

Though the muscle is doing a negative amount of mechanical work, (work is being done *on* the muscle), chemical energy (in fat, glucose or ATP) is nevertheless consumed, although less than would be consumed during a concentric contraction of the same force. For example, one expends more energy going up a flight of stairs than going down the same flight.

Muscles undergoing heavy eccentric loading suffer greater damage when overloaded (such as during muscle building or strength training exercise) as compared to concentric loading. When eccentric contractions are used in weight training, they are normally called *negatives*. During a concentric contraction, muscle fibers slide across each other, pulling the Z-lines together. During an eccentric contraction, the filaments slide past each other the opposite way, though the actual movement of the myosin heads during an eccentric contraction is not known. Exercise featuring a heavy eccentric load can actually support a greater weight (muscles are approximately 40% stronger during eccentric contractions than during concentric contractions) and also results in greater muscular damage and delayed onset muscle soreness one to two days after training. Exercise that incorporates both eccentric and concentric muscular contractions (i.e., involving a strong contraction and a controlled lowering of the weight) can produce greater gains in strength than concentric contractions alone. While unaccustomed heavy eccentric contractions can easily lead to overtraining, moderate training may confer protection against injury.

Eccentric Contractions in Movement

Eccentric contractions normally occur as a braking force in opposition to a concentric contraction to protect joints from damage. During virtually any routine movement, eccentric contractions assist in keeping motions smooth, but can also slow rapid movements such as a punch or throw. Part of training for rapid movements such as pitching during baseball involves reducing eccentric braking allowing a greater power to be developed throughout the movement.

Eccentric contractions are being researched for their ability to speed rehabilitation of weak or injured tendons. Achilles tendinitis and patellar tendonitis (also known as jumper's knee or patellar tendonosis) have been shown to benefit from high-load eccentric contractions.

Vertebrate Animals

In vertebrate animals, there are three types of muscle tissues: skeletal, smooth, and cardiac. Skeletal muscle constitutes the majority of muscle mass in the body and is responsible for locomotor activity. Smooth muscle forms blood vessels, gastrointestinal tract, and other areas in the body that produce sustained contractions. Cardiac muscle make up the heart, which pumps blood. Skeletal and cardiac muscles are called striated muscle because of their striped appearance under a microscope, which is due to the highly organized alternating pattern of A bands and I bands.

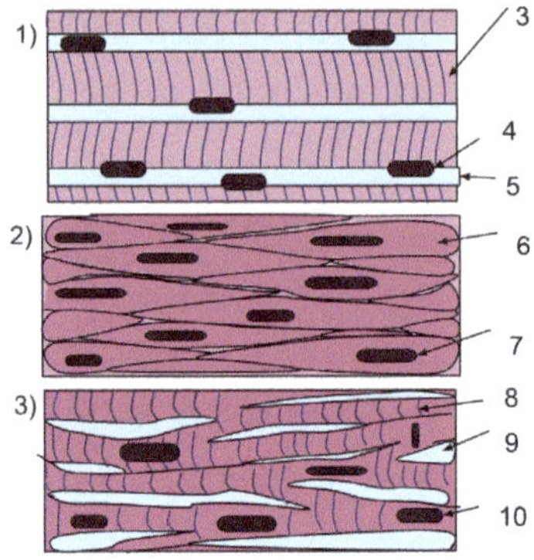

In vertebrate animals, there are three types of muscle tissues:
1) skeletal, 2) smooth, and 3) cardiac.

Skeletal Muscle

Excluding reflexes, all skeletal muscles contractions occur as a result of conscious effort originating in the brain. The brain sends electrochemical signals through the nervous system to the motor neuron that innervates several muscle fibers. In the case of some reflexes, the signal to contract can originate in the spinal cord through a feedback loop with the grey matter. Other actions such as locomotion, breathing, and chewing have a reflex aspect to them: the contractions can be initiated both consciously or unconsciously.

Neuromuscular Junction

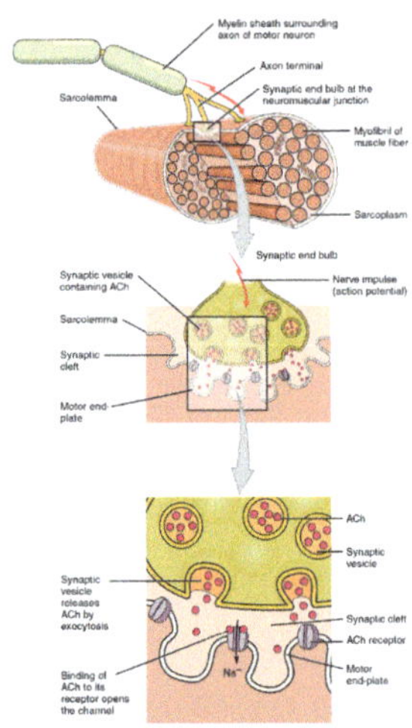

Structure of neuromuscular junction

A neuromuscular junction is a chemical synapse formed by the contact between a motor neuron and a muscle fiber. It is the site in which a motor neuron transmits a signal to a muscle fiber to initiate muscle contraction. The sequence of events that results in the depolarization of the muscle fiber at the neuromuscular junction begins when an action potential is initiated in the cell body of a motor neuron, which is then propagated by saltatory conduction along its axon toward the neuromuscular junction. Once it reaches the terminal bouton, the action potential causes a Ca^{2+} ion influx into the terminal by way of the voltage-gated calcium channels. The Ca^{2+} influx causes synaptic vesicles containing the neurotransmitter acetylcholine to fuse with the plasma membrane, releasing acetylcholine into the synaptic cleft between the motor neuron terminal and the neuromuscular junction of the skeletal muscle fiber. Acetylcholine diffuses across the synapse and binds to and activates nicotinic acetylcholine receptors on the neuromuscular junction. Activation of the nicotinic receptor opens its intrinsic sodium/potassium channel, causing sodium to rush in and potassium to trickle out. As a result, the sarcolemma reverses polarity and its voltage quickly jumps from the resting membrane potential of -90mV to as high as +75mV as sodium enters. The membrane potential then becomes hyperpolarized when potassium exits and is then adjusted back to the resting membrane potential. This rapid fluctuation is called the end-plate potential The voltage-gated ion channels of the sarcolemma next to the end plate open in response to the end plate potential. These voltage-gated channels are sodium and potassium specific and only allow one through. This wave of ion movements creates the action potential that spreads from the motor end plate in all directions. If action potentials stop arriving, then acetylcholine ceases to be released from the terminal bouton. The remaining acetylcholine in the synaptic cleft is either degraded by active acetylcholine esterase or reabsorbed by the synaptic knob and none is left to replace the degraded acetylcholine.

Excitation-contraction Coupling

Excitation–contraction coupling is the process by which a muscular action potential in the muscle fiber causes the myofibrils to contract. In skeletal muscle, excitation–contraction coupling relies on a direct coupling between key proteins, the sarcoplasmic reticulum (SR) calcium release channel (identified as the ryanodine receptor, RyR) and voltage-gated L-type calcium channels (identified as dihydropyridine receptors, DHPRs). DHPRs are located on the sarcolemma (which includes the surface sarcolemma and the transverse tubules), while the RyRs reside across the SR membrane. The close apposition of a transverse tubule and two SR regions containing RyRs is described as a triad and is predominantly where excitation–contraction coupling takes place. Excitation–contraction coupling occurs when depolarization of skeletal muscle cell results in a muscle action potential, which spreads across the cell surface and into the muscle fiber's network of T-tubules, thereby depolarizing the inner portion of the muscle fiber. Depolarization of the inner portions activates dihydropyridine receptors in the terminal cisternae, which are in close proximity to ryanodine receptors in the adjacent sarcoplasmic reticulum. The activated dihydropyridine receptors physically interact with ryanodine receptors to activate them via foot processes (involving conformational changes that allosterically activates the ryanodine receptors). As the ryanodine receptors open, Ca^{2+} is released from the sarcoplasmic reticulum into the local junctional space, which then diffuses into the bulk cytoplasm to cause a calcium spark. The sarcoplasmic reticulum has a large calcium buffering capacity partially due to a calcium-binding protein called calsequestrin. The near synchronous activation of thousands of calcium sparks by the action potential causes a cell-wide increase in calcium giving rise to the upstroke of the calcium transient. The Ca^{2+} released into the cytosol binds to Troponin C by the actin filaments, to allow crossbridge cycling, producing force and, in some situations, motion. The sarco/endoplasmic reticulum calcium-ATPase (SERCA) actively pumps Ca^{2+} back into the sarcoplasmic reticulum. As Ca^{2+} declines back to resting levels, the force declines and relaxation occurs.

Sliding Filament Theory

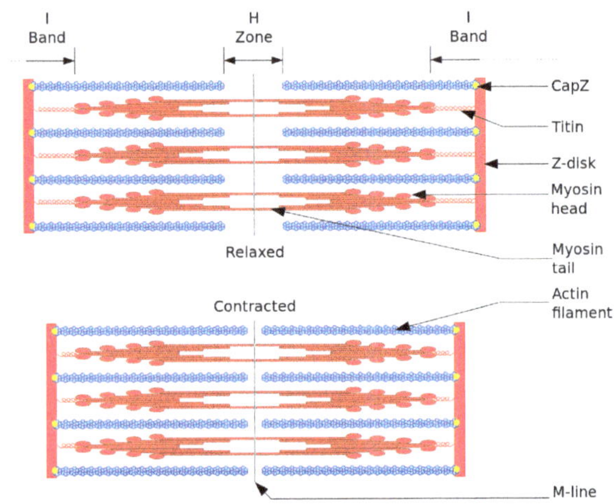

Sliding filament theory: A sarcomere in relaxed (above) and contracted (below) positions.

The sliding filament theory describes a process used by muscles to contract. It is a cycle of repetitive events that cause a thin filament to slide over a thick filament and generate tension in the muscle. It was independently developed by Andrew Huxley and Rolf Niedergerke and by Hugh Huxley and Jean Hanson in 1954. Physiologically, this contraction is not uniform across the sarcomere; the central position of the thick filaments becomes unstable and can shift during contraction. However the actions of elastic proteins such as titin are hypothesised to maintain uniform tension across the sarcomere and pull the thick filament into a central position.

Crossbridge Cycling

Crossbridge cycling is a sequence of molecular events that underlies the sliding filament theory. A crossbridge is a myosin projection, consisting of two myosin heads, that extends from the thick filaments. Each myosin head has two binding sites: one for ATP and another for actin. The binding of ATP to a myosin head detaches myosin from actin, thereby allowing myosin to bind to another actin molecule. Once attached, the ATP is hydrolyzed by myosin, which uses the released energy to move into the "cocked position" whereby it binds weakly to a part of the actin binding site. The remainder of the actin binding site is blocked by tropomyosin. With the ATP hydrolyzed, the cocked myosin head now contains ADP + P_i. Two Ca ions bind to troponin C on the actin filaments. The troponin $-Ca^{2+}$ complex causes tropomyosin to slide over and unblock the remainder of the actin binding site. Unblocking the rest of the actin binding sites allows the two myosin heads to close and myosin to bind strongly to actin. The myosin head then releases the inorganic phosphate and initiates a *power stroke,* which generates a force of 2 pN. The power stroke moves the actin filament inwards, thereby shortening the sarcomere. Myosin then releases ADP but still remains tightly bound to actin. At the end of the power stroke, ADP is released from the myosin head, leaving myosin attached to actin in a rigor state until another ATP binds to myosin. A lack of ATP would result in the rigor state characteristic of rigor mortis. Once another ATP binds to myosin, the myosin head will again detach from actin and another crossbridges cycle occurs.

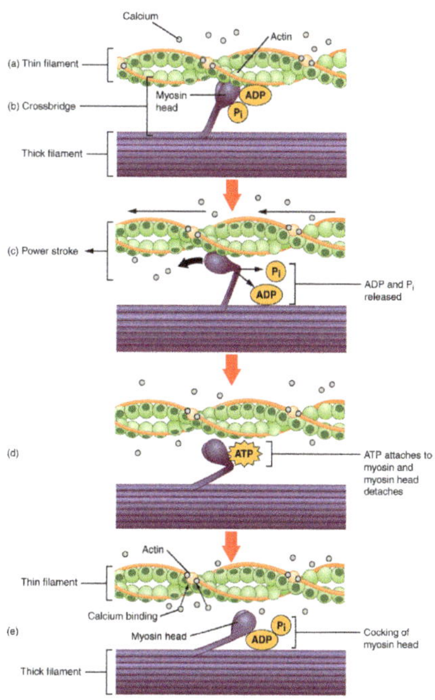

Crossbridge cycling

Crossbridge cycling is able to continue as long as there are sufficient amounts of ATP and Ca^{2+} in the cytoplasm. Termination of crossbridge cycling can occur when Ca^{2+} is actively pumped back into the sarcoplasmic reticulum. When Ca^{2+} is no longer present on the thin filament, the tropomyosin changes conformation back to its previous state so as to block the binding sites again. The myosin ceases binding to the thin filament, and the muscle relaxes. The Ca^{2+} ions leave the troponin molecule in order to maintain the Ca^{2+} ion concentration in the sarcoplasm. The active pumping of Ca^{2+} ions into the sarcoplasmic reticulum creates a deficiency in the fluid around the myofibrils. This causes the removal of Ca^{2+} ions from the troponin. Thus, the tropomyosin-troponin complex again covers the binding sites on the actin filaments and contraction ceases.

Gradation of Skeletal Muscle Contractions

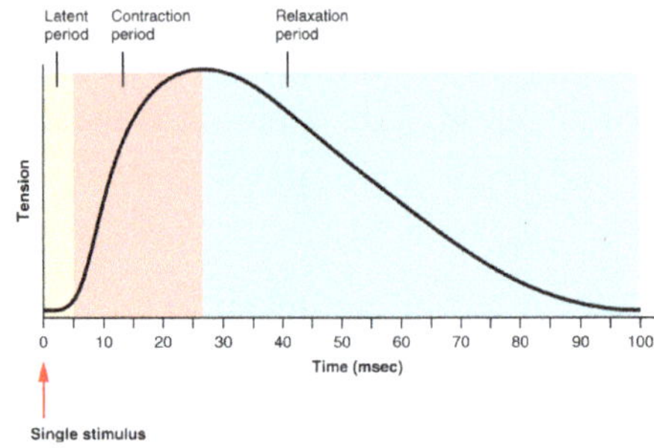

Twitch

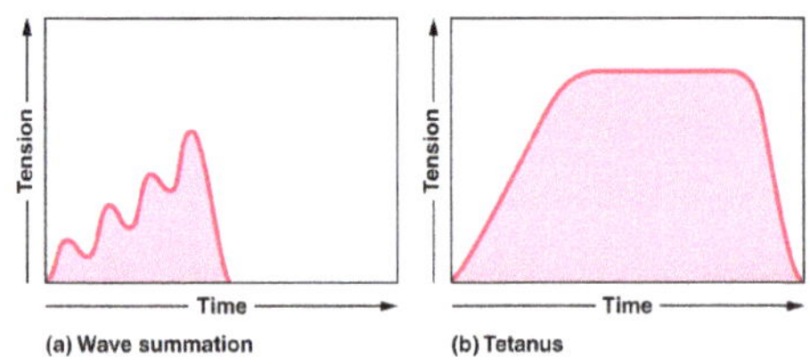

Summation and tetanus

Three Types of Skeletal Muscle Contractions

The strength of skeletal muscle contractions can be broadly separated into twitch, summation, and tetanus. A twitch is a single contraction and relaxation cycle produced by an action potential within the muscle fiber itself. The time between a stimulus to the motor nerve and the subsequent contraction of the innervated muscle is called the latent period, which usually takes about 10 ms and is caused by the time taken for nerve action potential to propagate, the time for chemical transmission at the neuromuscular junction, then the subsequent steps in excitation-contraction coupling.

If another muscle action potential were to be produced before the complete relaxation of a muscle twitch, then the next twitch will simply sum onto the previous twitch, thereby producing a *summation*. Summation can be achieved in two ways: *frequency summation* and *multiple fiber summation*. In frequency summation, the force exerted by the skeletal muscle is controlled by varying the frequency at which action potentials are sent to muscle fibers. Action potentials do not arrive at muscles synchronously, and, during a contraction, some fraction of the fibers in the muscle will be firing at any given time. In a typical circumstance, when a human is exerting a muscle as hard as he/she is consciously able, roughly one-third of the fibers in that muscle will be firing at once, though this ratio can be affected by various physiological and psychological factors (including Golgi tendon organs and Renshaw cells). This 'low' level of contraction is a protective mechanism to prevent avulsion of the tendon—the force generated by a 95% contraction of all fibers is sufficient to damage the body. In multiple fiber summation, if the central nervous system sends a weak signal to contract a muscle, the smaller motor units, being more excitable than the larger ones, are stimulated first. As the strength of the signal increases, more motor units are excited in addition to larger ones, with the largest motor units having as much as 50 times the contractile strength as the smaller ones. As more and larger motor units are activated, the force of muscle contraction becomes progressively stronger. A concept known as the size principle, allows for a gradation of muscle force during weak contraction to occur in small steps, which then become progressively larger when greater amounts of force are required.

Finally, if the frequency of muscle action potentials increases such that the muscle contraction reaches its peak force and plateaus at this level, then the contraction is a *tetanus*.

Length-tension Relationship

Length-tension relationship relates the strength of an isometric contraction to the length of the muscle at which the contraction occurs. Muscles operate with greatest active tension when close to an ideal length (often their resting length). When stretched or shortened beyond this (whether due to the action of the muscle itself or by an outside force), the maximum active tension generated decreases. This decrease is minimal for small deviations, but the tension drops off rapidly as the length deviates further from the ideal. Due to the presence of elastic proteins within a muscle cell (such as titin) and extracellular matrix, as the muscle is stretched beyond a given length, there is an entirely passive tension, which opposes lengthening. Combined together, there is a strong resistance to lengthening an active muscle far beyond the peak of active tension.

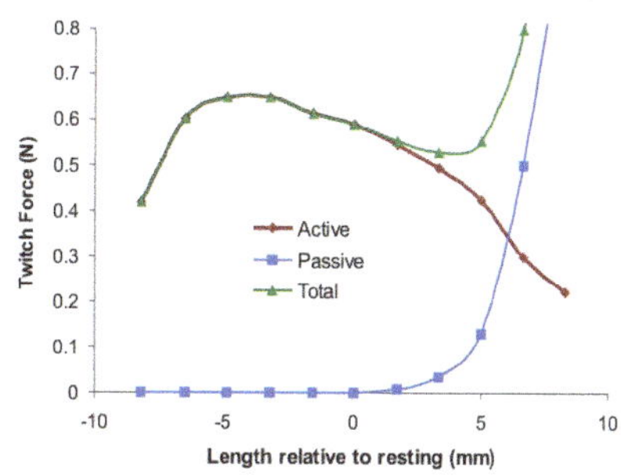

Muscle length versus isometric force

Force-velocity Relationships

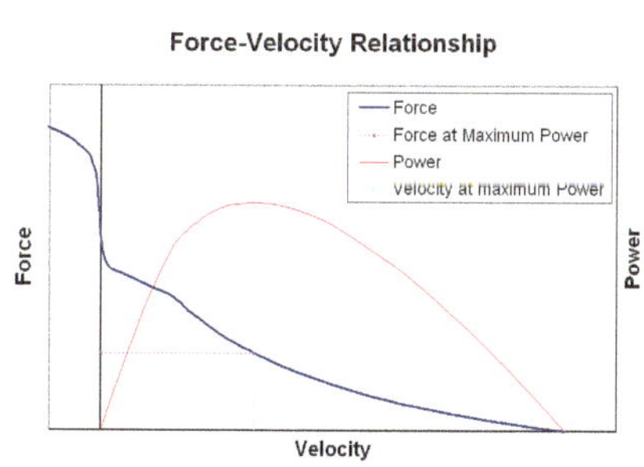

Force–velocity relationship: right of the vertical axis concentric contractions (the muscle is shortening), left of the axis eccentric contractions (the muscle is lengthened under load); power developed by the muscle in red.

Force–velocity relationship relates the speed at which a muscle changes its length (usually regulated by external forces, such as load or other muscles) to the amount of force that it generates. Force declines in a hyperbolic fashion relative to the isometric force as the shortening velocity increases, eventually reaching zero at some maximum velocity. The reverse holds true for when the muscle is stretched – force increases above isometric maximum, until finally reaching an absolute maximum. This has strong implications for the rate at which muscles can perform mechanical work (power). Since power is equal to force times velocity, the muscle generates no power at either isometric force (due to zero velocity) or maximal velocity (due to zero force). Instead, the optimal shortening velocity for power generation is approximately one-third of maximum shortening velocity.

These two fundamental properties of muscle have numerous biomechanical consequences, including limiting running speed, strength, and jumping distance and height.

Smooth Muscle

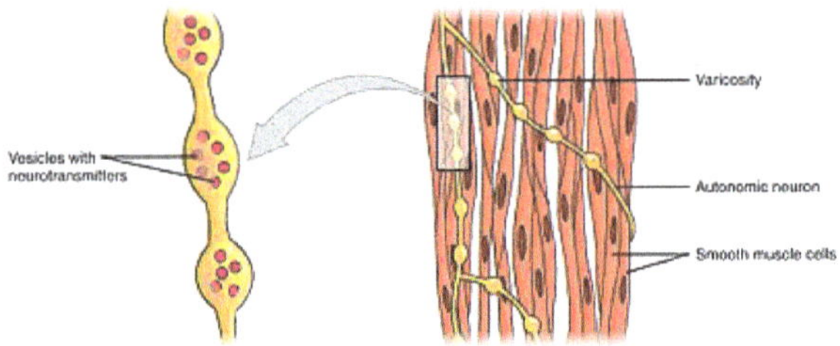

Swellings called varicosities belonging to an autonomic neuron innervate the smooth muscle cells.

Smooth muscles can be divided into two subgroups: single-unit (unitary) and multiunit. Single-unit smooth muscle cells can be found in the gut and blood vessels. Because these cells are linked together by gap junctions, they are able to contract as a syncytium. Single-unit smooth muscle cells contract myogenically, which can be modulated by the autonomic nervous system.

Unlike single-unit smooth muscle cells, multi-unit smooth muscle cells are found in the muscle of the eye and in the base of hair follicles. Multi-unit smooth muscle cells contract by being separately stimulated by nerves of the autonomic nervous system. As such, they allow for fine control and gradual responses, much like motor unit recruitment in skeletal muscle.

Mechanisms of Smooth Muscle Contraction

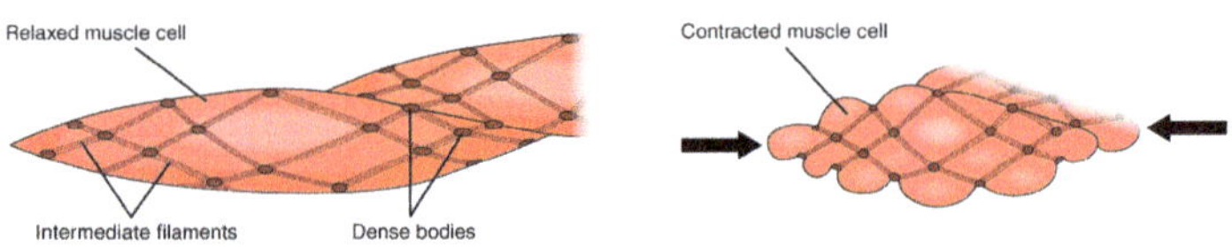

Smooth muscle contractions

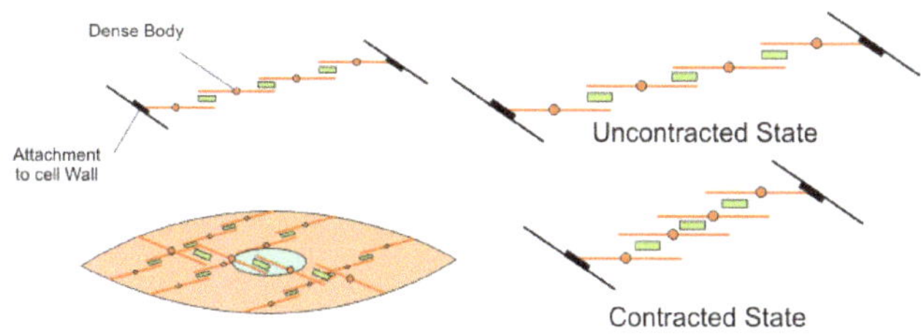

Actin-myosin filaments

Sliding filaments in contracted and uncontracted states

The contractile activity of smooth muscle cells is influenced by multiple inputs such as spontaneous electrical activity, neural and hormonal inputs, local changes in chemical composition, and stretch. This is in contrast to the contractile activity of skeletal muscle cells, which relies on a single neural input. Some types of smooth muscle cells are able to generate their own action potentials spontaneously, which usually occur following a pacemaker potential or a slow wave potential. These action potentials are generated by the influx of extracellular Ca^{2+}, and not Na^{+}. Like skeletal muscles, cytosolic Ca^{2+} ions are also required for crossbridge cycling in smooth muscle cells.

The two sources for cytosolic Ca^{2+} in smooth muscle cells are the extracellular Ca^{2+} entering through calcium channels and the Ca^{2+} ions that are released from the sarcoplasmic reticulum. The elevation of cytosolic Ca^{2+} results in more Ca^{2+} binding to calmodulin, which then binds and activates myosin light-chain kinase. The calcium-calmodulin-myosin light-chain kinase complex phosphorylates myosin on the 20 kilodalton (kDa) myosin light chains on amino acid residue-serine 19, initiating contraction and activating the myosin ATPase. Unlike skeletal muscle cells, smooth muscle cells lack troponin, even though they contain the thin filament protein tropomyosin and other notable proteins – caldesmon and calponin. Thus, smooth muscle contractions are initiated by the Ca^{2+} -activated phosphorylation of myosin rather than Ca^{2+} binding to the troponin complex that regulates myosin binding sites on actin like in skeletal and cardiac muscles.

Termination of crossbridge cycling (and leaving the muscle in latch-state) occurs when myosin light chain phosphatase removes the phosphate groups from the myosin heads. Phosphorylation of the 20 kDa myosin light chains correlates well with the shortening velocity of smooth muscle. During this period, there is a rapid burst of energy utilization as measured by oxygen consumption. Within a few minutes of initiation, the calcium level markedly decreases, the 20 kDa myosin light chains' phosphorylation decreases, and energy utilization decreases; however, force in tonic smooth muscle is maintained. During contraction of muscle, rapidly cycling crossbridges form between activated actin and phosphorylated myosin, generating force. It is hypothesized that the maintenance of force results from dephosphorylated "latch-bridges" that slowly cycle and maintain force. A number of kinases such as rho kinase, ZIP kinase, and protein kinase C are believed to participate in the sustained phase of contraction, and Ca flux may be significant.

Neuromodulation

Although smooth muscle contractions are myogenic, the rate and strength of their contractions can be modulated by the autonomic nervous system. Postganglionic nerve fibers of parasympathetic nervous system release the neurotransmitter acetylcholine, which binds to muscarinic acetylcholine receptors (mAChRs) on smooth muscle cells. These receptors are metabotropic, or G-protein coupled receptors that initiate a second messenger cascade. Conversely, postganglionic nerve fibers of the sympathetic nervous system release the neurotransmitters epinephrine and norepinephrine, which bind to adrenergic receptors that are also metabotropic. The exact effects on the smooth muscle depend on the specific characteristics of the receptor activated—both parasympathetic input and sympathetic input can be either excitatory (contractile) or inhibitory (relaxing).

Cardiac Muscle

There are two types of cardiac muscle cells: autorhythmic and contractile. Autorhythmic muscle cells do not contract, but instead set the pace of contraction for other cardiac muscle cells, which can be modulated by the autonomic nervous system. In contrast, contractile muscle cells constitute the majority of the heart muscle and are able to contract.

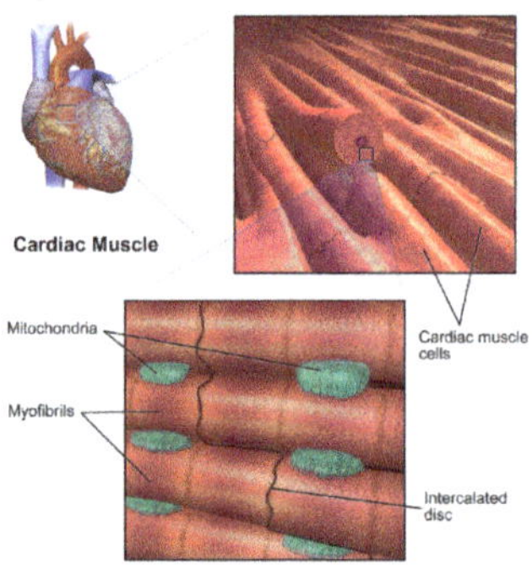

Cardiac muscle

Excitation-contraction Coupling

Unlike skeletal muscle, excitation–contraction coupling in cardiac muscle is thought to depend primarily on a mechanism called calcium-induced calcium release. Though the proteins involved are similar, the DHPR and RyR (type 2) are not physically coupled. Instead, RyRs are activated by a calcium trigger, which is brought about by the activation of DHPRs. Further, cardiac muscle tend to exhibit diad (or dyad) structures, rather than triads.

Excitation-contraction coupling in cardiac muscle cells occurs when an action potential is initiated by pacemaker cells in the Sinoatrial node or Atrioventricular node and conducted to all cells in the heart via gap junctions. The action potential travels along the surface membrane into T-tubules (the latter are not seen in all cardiac cell types) and the depolarisation causes extracellular Ca^{2+} to enter the cell via L-type calcium channels and possibly sodium-calcium exchanger during the early part of the plateau phase. This Ca^{2+} influx causes a small local increase in intracellular Ca^{2+}. The increase in Ca^{2+} is detected by ryanodine receptors in the membrane of the sarcoplasmic reticulum which releases Ca^{2+} in a positive feedback physiological response. This positive feedback is known as calcium-induced calcium release and gives rise to calcium sparks (Ca^{2+} sparks). The spatial and temporal summation of ~30,000 Ca^{2+} sparks gives a cell-wide increase in cytoplasmic calcium concentration. The cytoplasmic calcium binds to Troponin C, moving the tropomyosin complex off the actin binding site allowing the myosin head to bind to the actin filament. From this point on, the contractile mechanism is essentially the same as for skeletal muscle (above). Briefly, using ATP hydrolysis, the myosin head pulls the actin filament toward the centre of the sarcomere. Intracellular calcium is taken up by the sarco/endoplasmic reticulum ATPase pump back into the sarcoplasmic reticulum ready for the next cycle to begin. Calcium is also ejected from the cell mainly by the sodium-calcium exchanger and, to a lesser extent, a plasma membrane calcium ATPase and/or taken up by the mitochondria. An enzyme, phospholamban, serves as a brake for the ATPase. At low heart rates, phospholamban is active and slows down the activity of the ATPase so that Ca^{2+} does not have to leave the cell entirely. At high heart rates, phospholamban is phosphorylated and deactivated thus removing most Ca^{2+} from the cell back into the sarcoplasmic reticulum. This allows the heart muscles to relax to allow for ventricular filling. Intracellular calcium concentration drops and troponin complex returns over the active site of the actin filament, ending contraction.

Invertebrate Animals

Circular and Longitudinal Muscles

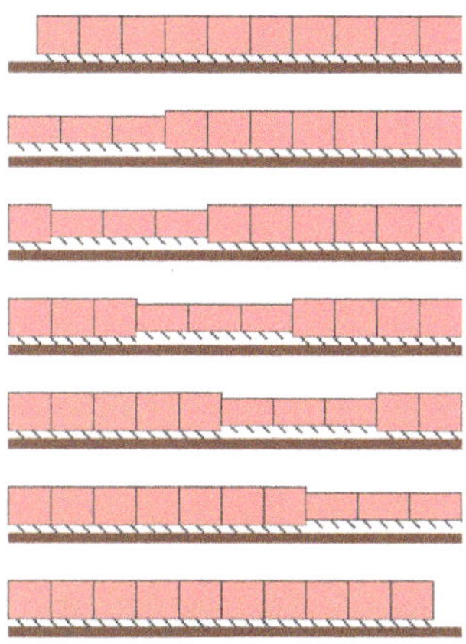

A simplified image showing earthworm movement via peristalsis

In annelids such as earthworms and leeches, circular and longitudinal muscles cells form the body wall of these animals and are responsible for their movement. In an earthworm that is moving through a soil, for example, contractions of circular and longitudinal muscles occur reciprocally while the coelomic fluid serves as a hydroskeleton by maintaining turgidity of the earthworm. When the circular muscles in the anterior segments contract, the anterior portion of animal's body begins to constrict radially, which pushes the incompressible coelomic fluid forward and increasing the length of the animal. As a result, the front end of the animal moves forward. As the front end of the earthworm becomes anchored and the circular muscles in the anterior segments become relaxed, a wave of longitudinal muscle contractions passes backwards, which pulls the rest of animal's trailing body forward. These alternating waves of circular and longitudinal contractions is called peristalsis, which underlies the creeping movement of earthworms.

Obliquely Striated Muscles

Invertebrates such as annelids, mollusks, and nematodes, possess obliquely striated muscles, which contain bands of thick and thin filaments that are arranged helically rather than transversely, like in vertebrate skeletal or cardiac muscles. In bivalves, the obliquely striated muscles can maintain tension over long periods without using too much energy. Bivalves use these muscles to keep their shells closed.

Asynchronous Muscles

Advanced insects such as wasps, flies, bees, and beetles possess asynchronous muscles that constitute the flight muscles in these animals. These flight muscles are often called *fibrillar muscles* because they contain myofibrils that are thick and conspicuous. A remarkable feature of these muscles is that they do not require stimulation for each muscle contraction. Hence, they are called *asynchronous muscles* because the number of contractions in these muscles do not correspond (or synchronize) with the number of action potentials. For example, a wing muscle of a tethered fly may receive action potentials at a frequency of 3 Hz but it is able to beat at a frequency of 120 Hz. The high frequency beating is made possible because the muscles are connected to a resonant system, which is driven to a natural frequency of vibration.

History

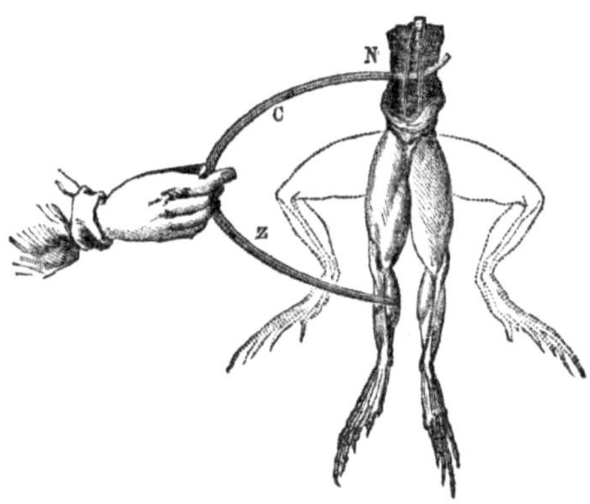

Electrodes touch a frog, and the legs twitch into the upward position

In 1780, Luigi Galvani discovered that the muscles of dead frogs' legs twitched when struck by an electrical spark. This was one of the first forays into the study of bioelectricity, a field that still studies the electrical patterns and signals in tissues such as nerves and muscles.

In 1952, the term excitation–contraction coupling was coined to describe the physiological process of converting an electrical stimulus to a mechanical response. This process is fundamental to muscle physiology, whereby the electrical stimulus is usually an action potential and the mechanical response is contraction. Excitation–contraction coupling can be dysregulated in many diseases.Though excitation–contraction coupling has been known for over half a century, it is still an active area of biomedical research. The general scheme is that an action potential arrives to depolarize the cell membrane. By mechanisms specific to the muscle type, this depolarization results in an increase in cytosolic calcium that is called a calcium transient. This increase in calcium activates calcium-sensitive contractile proteins that then use ATP to cause cell shortening.

The mechanism for muscle contraction evaded scientists for years and requires continued research and updating. The sliding filament theory was independently developed by Andrew F. Huxley and Rolf Niedergerke and by Hugh Huxley and Jean Hanson. Their findings were published as two consecutive papers published in the 22 May 1954 issue of *Nature* under the common theme "Structural Changes in Muscle During Contraction".

Isotonic Contraction

In an isotonic contraction, tension remains the same, whilst the muscle's length changes. Isotonic contractions differ from isokinetic contractions in that in isokinetic contractions the muscle speed remains constant. While superficially identical, as the muscle's force changes via the length-tension relationship during a contraction, an isotonic contraction will keep force constant while velocity changes, but an isokinetic contraction will keep velocity constant while force changes. A near isotonic contraction is known as Auxotonic contraction.

There are two types of isotonic contractions: (1) concentric and (2) eccentric. In a concentric contraction, the muscle tension rises to meet the resistance, then remains the same as the muscle shortens. In eccentric, the muscle lengthens due to the resistance being greater than the force the muscle is producing.

Concentric

This type is typical of most exercise. The external force on the muscle is less than the force the muscle is generating - a *shortening* contraction. The effect is not visible during the classic biceps curl, which is in fact auxotonic because the resistance (torque due to the weight being lifted) does not remain the same through the exercise. Tension is highest at a parallel to the floor level, and eases off above and below this point. Therefore, tension changes as well as muscle length.

Eccentric

There are two main features to note regarding eccentric contractions. First, the absolute tensions achieved can be very high relative to the muscle's maximum tetanic tension generating capacity (you can set down a much heavier object than you can lift). Second, the absolute tension is relatively independent of lengthening velocity.

Muscle injury and soreness are selectively associated with eccentric contraction. Muscle strengthening using exercises that involve eccentric contractions is lower than using concentric exercises. However because higher levels of tension are easier to attain during exercises that involve eccentric contractions it may be that, by generating higher signals for muscle strengthening, muscle hypertrophy is better than exercises that involve concentric contractions, albeit at a higher level of resistance.

Auxotonic Contraction

This is almost an isotonic contraction because there is some fluctuation towards the end of the contraction. For example, the heart's ventricles contract to expel blood into the pulmonary artery and aorta. As the blood flows out, the previous built-up load is decreased and hence less force is required to expel the rest of the blood. Thus the tension is reduced.

Tendon

A tendon or sinew is a tough band of fibrous connective tissue that usually connects muscle to bone and is capable of withstanding tension.

Tendons are similar to ligaments; both are made of collagen. Ligaments join one bone to another bone, while tendons connect muscle to bone.

Structure

Histologically, tendons consist of dense regular connective tissue fascicles encased in dense irregular connective tissue sheaths. Normal healthy tendons are composed mostly of parallel arrays of collagen fibers closely packed together. The dry mass of normal tendons, which makes up about 30% of their total mass, is composed of about 86% collagen, 2% elastin, 1–5% proteoglycans, and 0.2% inorganic components such as copper, manganese, and calcium. The collagen portion is made up of 97–98% type I collagen, with small amounts of other types of collagen. These include type II collagen in the cartilaginous zones, type III collagen in the reticulin fibres of the vascular walls, type IX collagen, type IV collagen in the basement membranes of the capillaries, type V collagen in the vascular walls, and type X collagen in the mineralized fibrocartilage near the interface with the bone. Collagen fibres coalesce into macroaggregates. After secretion from the cell, the terminal peptides are cleaved by procollagen N- and C-proteinases, and the tropocollagen molecules spontaneously assemble into insoluble fibrils. A collagen molecule is about 300 nm long and 1–2 nm wide, and the diameter of the fibrils that are formed can range from 50–500 nm. In tendons, the fibrils then assemble further to form fascicles, which are about 10 mm in length with a diameter of 50–300 μm, and finally into a tendon fibre with a diameter of 100–500 μm. Fascicles are bound by the endotendineum, which is a delicate loose connective tissue containing thin collagen fibrils. and elastic fibres. Groups of fascicles are bounded by the epitenon. Filling the interstitia within the fascia where the tendon is located is the paratenon a fatty areolar tissue.

The collagen in tendons are held together with proteoglycan components including decorin and, in compressed regions of tendon, aggrecan, which are capable of binding to the collagen fibrils at specific locations. The proteoglycans are interwoven with the collagen fibrils – their glycosaminoglycan (GAG) side chains have multiple interactions with the surface of the fibrils – showing that the proteoglycans are important structurally in the interconnection of the fibrils. The major GAG components of the tendon are dermatan sulfate and chondroitin sulfate, which associate with collagen and are involved in the fibril assembly process during tendon development. Dermatan sulfate is thought to be responsible for forming associations between fibrils, while chondroitin sulfate is thought to be more involved with occupying volume between the fibrils to keep them separated and help withstand deformation. The dermatan sulfate side chains of decorin aggregate in solution, and this behavior can assist with the assembly of the collagen fibrils. When decorin molecules are bound to a collagen fibril, their dermatan sulfate chains may extend and associate with other dermatan sulfate chains on decorin that is bound to separate fibrils, therefore creating interfibrillar bridges and eventually causing parallel alignment of the fibrils.

The tenocytes produce the collagen molecules, which aggregate end-to-end and side-to-side to produce collagen fibrils. Fibril bundles are organized to form fibres with the elongated tenocytes closely packed between them. There is a three-dimensional network of cell processes associated with collagen in the tendon. The cells communicate with each other through gap junctions, and this signalling gives them the ability to detect and respond to mechanical loading.

Blood vessels may be visualized within the endotendon running parallel to collagen fibres, with occasional branching transverse anastomoses.

The internal tendon bulk is thought to contain no nerve fibres, but the epitenon and paratenon contain nerve endings, while Golgi tendon organs are present at the junction between tendon and muscle.

Tendon length varies in all major groups and from person to person. Tendon length is, in practice, the deciding factor regarding actual and potential muscle size. For example, all other relevant biological factors being equal, a man with a shorter tendons and a longer biceps muscle will have greater potential for muscle mass than a man with a longer tendon and a shorter muscle. Successful bodybuilders will generally have shorter tendons. Conversely, in sports requiring athletes to excel in actions such as running or jumping, it is beneficial to have longer than average Achilles tendon and a shorter calf muscle.

Tendon length is determined by genetic predisposition, and has not been shown to either increase or decrease in response to environment, unlike muscles, which can be shortened by trauma, use imbalances and a lack of recovery and stretching.

Functions

Traditionally, tendons have been considered to be a mechanism by which muscles connect to bone, functioning to transmit forces. This connection allows tendons to passively modulate forces during locomotion, providing additional stability with no active work. However, over the past two decades, much research focused on the elastic properties of some tendons and their ability to function as springs. Not all tendons are required to perform the same functional role, with some predominantly positioning limbs, such as the fingers when writing (positional tendons) and others acting as springs to make locomotion more efficient (energy storing tendons). Energy storing tendons can store and recover energy at high efficiency. For example, during a human stride, the Achilles tendon stretches as the ankle joint dorsiflexes. During the last portion of the stride, as the foot plantar-flexes (pointing the toes down), the stored elastic energy is released. Furthermore, because the tendon stretches, the muscle is able to function with less or even no change in length, allowing the muscle to generate greater force.

The mechanical properties of the tendon are dependent on the collagen fiber diameter and orientation. The collagen fibrils are parallel to each other and closely packed, but show a wave-like appearance due to planar undulations, or crimps, on a scale of several micrometers. In tendons, the collagen fibres have some flexibility due to the absence of hydroxyproline and proline residues at specific locations in the amino acid sequence, which allows the formation of other conformations such as bends or internal loops in the triple helix and results in the development of crimps. The crimps in the collagen fibrils allow the tendons to have some flexibility as well as a low compressive stiffness. In addition, because the tendon is a multi-stranded structure made up of many partially independent fibrils and fascicles, it does not behave as a single rod, and this property also contributes to its flexibility.

The proteoglycan components of tendons also are important to the mechanical properties. While the collagen fibrils allow tendons to resist tensile stress, the proteoglycans allow them to resist compressive stress. These molecules are very hydrophilic, meaning that they can absorb a large amount of water and therefore have a high swelling ratio. Since they are noncovalently bound to the fibrils, they may reversibly associate and disassociate so that the bridges between fibrils can be broken and reformed. This process may be involved in allowing the fibril to elongate and decrease in diameter under tension. However, the proteoglycans may also have a role in the tensile properties of tendon. The structure of tendon is effectively a fibre composite material, built as a series of hierarchical levels. At each level of the hierarchy, the collagen units are bound together by either collagen crosslinks, or the proteoglycans, to create a structure highly resistant to tensile load. The elongation and the strain of the collagen fibrils alone have been shown to be much lower than the total elongation and strain of the entire tendon under the same amount of stress, demonstrating that the proteoglycan-rich matrix must also undergo deformation, and stiffening of the matrix occurs at high strain rates. This deformation of the non-collagenous matrix occurs at all levels of the tendon hierarchy, and by modulating the organisation and structure of this matrix, the different mechanical properties required by different tendons can be achieved. Energy storing tendons have been shown to utilise significant amounts of sliding between fascicles to enable the high strain characteristics they require, whilst positional tendons rely more heavily on sliding between collagen fibres and fibrils. However, recent data suggests that energy storing tendons may also contain fascicles which are twisted, or helical, in nature - an arrangement that would be highly beneficial for providing the spring-like behaviour required in these tendons.

Mechanics

Tendons are viscoelastic structures, which means they exhibit both elastic and viscous behaviour. When stretched, tendons exhibit typical "soft tissue" behavior. The force-extension, or stress-strain curve starts with a very low stiffness region, as the crimp structure straightens and the collagen fibres align suggesting negative Poisson's ratio in the fibres of the tendon. More recently, tests carried out in vivo (through MRI) and ex vivo (through mechanical testing of various cadaveric tendon tissue) have shown that healthy tendons are highly anisotropic and exhibit a negative Poisson's ratio (auxetic) in some planes when stretched up to 2% along their length, i.e. within their normal range of motion. After this 'toe' region, the structure becomes significantly stiffer, and has a linear stress-strain curve until it begins to fail. The mechanical properties of tendons vary widely, as they are matched to the functional requirements of the tendon. The energy storing tendons tend to be more elastic, or less stiff, so they can more easily store energy, whilst the stiffer positional tendons tend to be a little more viscoelastic, and less elastic, so they can provide finer control of movement. A typical energy storing tendon will fail at around 12-15% strain, and a stress in the region of 100-150 MPa, although some tendons are notably more extensible than this, for example the superficial digital flexor in the horse, which stretches in excess of 20% when galloping. Positional tendons can fail at strains as low as 6-8%, but can have moduli in the region of 700-1000 MPa.

Several studies have demonstrated that tendons respond to changes in mechanical loading with growth and remodeling processes, much like bones. In particular, a study showed that disuse of the Achilles tendon in rats resulted in a decrease in the average thickness of the collagen fiber bundles comprising the tendon. In humans, an experiment in which people were subjected to a simulated micro-gravity environment found that tendon stiffness decreased significantly, even when subjects were required to perform restiveness exercises. These effects have implications in areas ranging from treatment of bedridden patients to the design of more effective exercises for astronauts.

Healing

The tendons in the foot are highly complex and intricate. Therefore, the healing process for a broken tendon is long and painful. Most people who do not receive medical attention within the first 48 hours of the injury will suffer from severe swelling, pain, and a burning sensation where the injury occurred.

It was believed previously that tendons could not undergo matrix turnover and that tenocytes were not capable of repair. However, it has been shown more recently that, throughout the lifetime of a person, tenocytes in the tendon actively synthesize ECM components as well as enzymes such as matrix metalloproteinases (MMPs) can degrade the matrix. Tendons are capable of healing and recovering from injuries in a process that is controlled by the tenocytes and their surrounding extracellular matrix.

The three main stages of tendon healing are inflammation, repair or proliferation, and remodeling, which can be further divided into consolidation and maturation. These stages can overlap with each other. In the first stage, inflammatory cells such as neutrophils are recruited to the injury site, along with erythrocytes. Monocytes and macrophages are recruited within the first 24 hours, and phagocytosis of necrotic materials at the injury site occurs. After the release of vasoactive and chemotactic factors, angiogenesis and the proliferation of tenocytes are initiated. Tenocytes then move into the site and start to synthesize collagen III. After a few days, the repair or proliferation stage begins. In this stage, the tenocytes are involved in the synthesis of large amounts of collagen and proteoglycans at the site of injury, and the levels of GAG and water are high. After about six weeks, the remodeling stage begins. The first part of this stage is consolidation, which lasts from about six to ten weeks after the injury. During this time, the synthesis of collagen and GAGs is decreased, and the cellularity is also decreased as the tissue becomes more fibrous as a result of increased production of collagen I and the fibrils become aligned in the direction of mechanical stress. The final maturation stage occurs after ten weeks, and during this time there is an increase in crosslinking of the collagen fibrils, which causes the tissue to become stiffer. Gradually, over about one year, the tissue will turn from fibrous to scar-like.

Matrix metalloproteinases or MMPs have a very important role in the degradation and remodeling of the ECM during the healing process after a tendon injury. Certain MMPs including MMP-1, MMP-2, MMP-8, MMP-13, and MMP-14 have collagenase activity, meaning that, unlike many other enzymes, they are capable of degrading collagen I fibrils. The degradation of the collagen fibrils by MMP-1 along with the presence of denatured collagen are factors that are believed to cause weakening of the tendon ECM and an increase in the potential for another rupture to occur. In response to repeated mechanical loading or injury, cytokines may be released by tenocytes and can induce the release of MMPs, causing degradation of the ECM and leading to recurring injury and chronic tendinopathies.

A variety of other molecules are involved in tendon repair and regeneration. There are five growth factors that have been shown to be significantly upregulated and active during tendon healing: insulin-like growth factor 1 (IGF-I), platelet-derived growth factor (PDGF), vascular endothelial growth factor (VEGF), basic fibroblast growth factor (bFGF), and transforming growth factor beta (TGF-β). These growth factors all have different roles during the healing process. IGF-1 increases collagen and proteoglycan production during the first stage of inflammation, and PDGF is also present during the early stages after injury and promotes the synthesis of other growth factors along with the synthesis of DNA and the proliferation of tendon cells. The three isoforms of TGF-β (TGF-β1, TGF-β2, TGF-β3) are known to play a role in wound healing and scar formation. VEGF is well known to promote angiogenesis and to induce endothelial cell proliferation and migration, and VEGF mRNA has been shown to be expressed at the site of tendon injuries along with collagen I mRNA. Bone morphogenetic proteins (BMPs) are a subgroup of TGF-β superfamily that can induce bone and cartilage formation as well as tissue differentiation, and BMP-12 specifically has been shown to influence formation and differentiation of tendon tissue and to promote fibrogenesis.

Effects of Activity on Healing

In animal models, extensive studies have been conducted to investigate the effects of mechanical strain in the form of activity level on tendon injury and healing. While stretching can disrupt healing during the initial inflammatory phase, it has been shown that controlled movement of the tendons after about one week following an acute injury can help to promote the synthesis of collagen by the tenocytes, leading to increased tensile strength and diameter of the healed tendons and fewer adhesions than tendons that are immobilized. In chronic tendon injuries, mechanical loading has also been shown to stimulate fibroblast proliferation and collagen synthesis along with collagen realignment, all of which promote repair and remodeling. To further support the theory that movement and activity assist in tendon healing, it has been shown that immobilization of the tendons after injury often has a negative effect on healing. In rabbits, collagen fascicles that are immobilized have shown decreased tensile strength, and immobilization also results in lower amounts of water, proteoglycans, and collagen crosslinks in the tendons.

Several mechanotransduction mechanisms have been proposed as reasons for the response of tenocytes to mechanical force that enable them to alter their gene expression, protein synthesis, and cell phenotype, and eventually cause changes in tendon structure. A major factor is mechanical deformation of the extracellular matrix, which can affect the actin cytoskeleton and therefore affect cell shape, motility, and function. Mechanical forces can be transmitted by focal adhesion sites, integrins, and cell-cell junctions. Changes in the actin cytoskeleton can activate integrins, which mediate "outside-in" and "inside-out" signaling between the cell and the matrix. G-proteins, which induce intracellular signaling cascades, may also be important, and ion channels are activated by stretching to allow ions such as calcium, sodium, or potassium to enter the cell.

Society and Culture

Sinew was widely used throughout pre-industrial eras as a tough, durable fiber. Some specific uses include using sinew as thread for sewing, attaching feathers to arrows, lashing tool blades to shafts, etc. It is also recommended in survival guides as a material from which strong cordage can be made for items like traps or living structures. Tendon must be treated in specific ways to function usefully for these purposes. Inuit and other circumpolar people utilized sinew as the only cordage for all domestic purposes due to the lack of other suitable fiber sources in their ecological habitats. The elastic properties of particular sinews were also used in composite recurved bows favoured by the steppe nomads of Eurasia. The first stone throwing artillery also used the elastic properties of sinew.

Sinew makes for an excellent cordage material for three reasons: It is extremely strong, it contains natural glues, and it shrinks as it dries, doing away with the need for knots.

Culinary uses

Tendon (in particular, beef tendon) is used as a food in some Asian cuisines (often served at yum cha or dim sum restaurants). One popular dish is *suan bao niu jin*, in which the tendon is marinated in garlic. It is also sometimes found in the Vietnamese noodle dish phở.

Clinical Significance

Injury

Tendons are subject to many types of injuries. There are various forms of tendinopathies or tendon injuries due to overuse. These types of injuries generally result in inflammation and degeneration or weakening of the tendons, which may eventually lead to tendon rupture. Tendinopathies can be caused by a number of factors relating to the tendon extracellular matrix (ECM), and their classification has been difficult because their symptoms and histopathology often are similar.

The first category of tendinopathy is paratenonitis, which refers to inflammation of the paratenon, or paratendinous sheet located between the tendon and its sheath. Tendinosis refers to non-inflammatory injury to the tendon at the cellular level. The degradation is caused by damage to collagen, cells, and the vascular components of the tendon, and is known to lead to rupture. Observations of tendons that have undergone spontaneous rupture have shown the presence of collagen fibrils that are not in the correct parallel orientation or are not uniform in length or diameter, along with rounded tenocytes, other cell abnormalities, and the ingrowth of blood vessels. Other forms of tendinosis that have not led to rupture have also shown the degeneration, disorientation, and thinning of the collagen fibrils, along with an increase in the amount of glycosaminoglycans between the fibrils. The third is paratenonitis with tendinosis, in which combinations of paratenon inflammation and tendon degeneration are both present. The last is tendinitis, which refers to degeneration with inflammation of the tendon as well as vascular disruption.

Tendinopathies may be caused by several intrinsic factors including age, body weight, and nutrition. The extrinsic factors are often related to sports and include excessive forces or loading, poor training techniques, and environmental conditions.

Other Animals

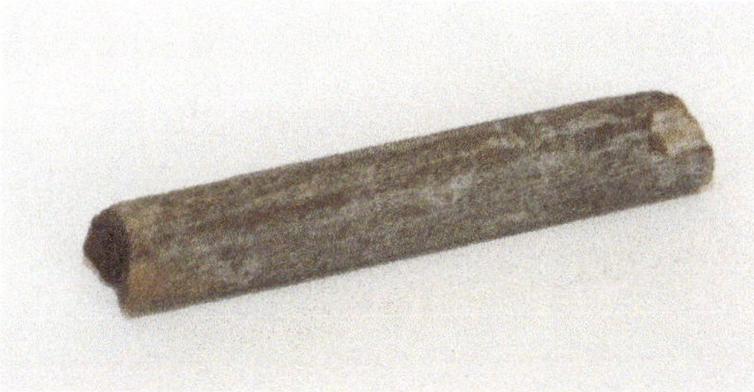

Ossified tendon from an Edmontosaurus bone bed in Wyoming (Lance Formation)

In some organisms, notable ones being birds and ornithischian dinosaurs, portions of the tendon can become ossified. In this process, osteocytes infiltrate the tendon and lay down bone as they would in sesamoid bone such as the patella. In birds, tendon ossification primarily occurs in the hindlimb, while in ornithischian dinosaurs, ossified axial muscle tendons form a latticework along the neural and haemal spines on the tail, presumably for support.

Joint

A joint or articulation (or articular surface) is the connection made between bones in the body which link the skeletal system into a functional whole. They are constructed to allow for different degrees and types of movement. Some joints, such as the knee, elbow, and shoulder, are self-lubricating, almost frictionless, and are able to withstand compression and maintain heavy loads while still executing smooth and precise movements. Other joints such as sutures between the bones of the skull permit very little movement (only during birth) in order to protect the brain and the sense organs. The connection between a tooth and the jawbone is also called a joint, and is described as a fibrous joint known as a gomphosis. Joints are classified both structurally and functionally.

Classification

Joints are mainly classified structurally and functionally. Structural classification is determined by how the bones connect to each other, while functional classification is determined by the degree of movement between the articulating bones. In practice, there is significant overlap between the two types of classifications.

Clinical, numerical Classification

- monoarticular – concerning one joint
- oligoarticular or pauciarticular – concerning 2–4 joints
- polyarticular – concerning 5 or more joints

Structural Classification (Binding Tissue)

Structural classification names and divides joints according to the type of binding tissue that connects the bones to each other. There are three structural classifications of joints:

- fibrous joint – joined by dense regular connective tissue that is rich in collagen fibers
- cartilaginous joint – joined by cartilage
- synovial joint – not directly joined – the bones have a synovial cavity and are united by the dense irregular connective tissue that forms the articular capsule that is normally associated with accessory ligaments.
- facet joint – joint between two articular processes between two vertebrae.

Functional Classification (Movement)

Joints can also be classified functionally according to the type and degree of movement they allow: Joint movements are described with reference to the basic anatomical planes.

- synarthrosis – permits little or no mobility. Most synarthrosis joints are fibrous joints (e.g., skull sutures).
- amphiarthrosis – permits slight mobility. Most amphiarthrosis joints are cartilaginous joints (e.g., intervertebral discs).
- synovial joint (also known as a *diarthrosis*) – freely movable. Synovial joints can in turn be classified into six groups according to the type of movement they allow: plane joint, ball and socket joint, hinge joint, pivot joint, condyloid joint and saddle joint.

Joints can also be classified, according to the number of axes of movement they allow, into nonaxial (gliding, as between the proximal ends of the ulna and radius), monoaxial (uniaxial), biaxial and multiaxial. Another classification is according to the degrees of freedom allowed, and distinguished between joints with one, two or three degrees of freedom. A further classification is according to the number and shapes of the articular surfaces: flat, concave and convex surfaces. Types of articular surfaces include trochlear surfaces.

Biomechanical Classification

Joints can also be classified based on their anatomy or on their biomechanical properties. According to the anatomic classification, joints are subdivided into *simple* and *compound*, depending on the number of bones involved, and into *complex* and *combination* joints:

1. Simple joint: two articulation surfaces (e.g. shoulder joint, hip joint)
2. Compound joint: three or more articulation surfaces (e.g. radiocarpal joint)
3. Complex joint: two or more articulation surfaces and an articular disc or meniscus (e.g. knee joint)

Anatomical

The joints may be classified anatomically into the following groups:

1. Joints of hand
2. Elbow joints
3. Wrist joints
4. Axillary articulations
5. Sternoclavicular joints
6. Vertebral articulations
7. Temporomandibular joints
8. Sacroiliac joints
9. Hip joints
10. Knee joints
11. Articulations of foot

Clinical Significance

Damaging the cartilage of joints (articular cartilage) or the bones and muscles that stabilize the joints can lead to joint dislocations and osteoarthritis. Swimming is a great way to exercise the joints with minimal damage.

A joint disorder is termed arthropathy, and when involving inflammation of one or more joints the disorder is called arthritis. Most joint disorders involve arthritis, but joint damage by external physical trauma is typically not termed arthritis.

Arthropathies are called *polyarticular* (multiarticular) when involving many joints and *monoarticular* when involving only a single joint.

Arthritis is the leading cause of disability in people over the age of 55. There are many different forms of arthritis, each of which has a different cause. The most common form of arthritis, osteoarthritis (also known as degenerative joint disease), occurs following trauma to the joint, following an infection of the joint or simply as a result of aging and the deterioration of articular cartilage. Furthermore, there is emerging evidence that abnormal anatomy may contribute to early development of osteoarthritis. Other forms of arthritis are rheumatoid arthritis and psoriatic arthritis, which are autoimmune diseases in which the body is attacking itself. Septic arthritis is caused by joint infection. Gouty arthritis is caused by deposition of uric acid crystals in the joint that results in subsequent inflammation. Additionally, there is a less common form of gout that is caused by the formation of rhomboidal-shaped crystals of calcium pyrophosphate. This form of gout is known as pseudogout.

Temporomandibular joint syndrome (TMJ) involves the jaw joints and can cause facial pain, clicking sounds in the jaw, or limitation of jaw movement, to name a few symptoms. It is caused by psychological tension and misalignment of the jaw (malocclusion), and may be affecting as many as 75 million Americans.

References

- Kier, William M. (2012-04-15). "The diversity of hydrostatic skeletons". Journal of Experimental Biology. 215 (8): 1247–1257. ISSN 0022-0949. PMID 22442361. doi:10.1242/jeb.056549
- Barnes, Edward E.; Fox, Richard S.; Barnes, Robert D. (2003). Invertebrate zoology : a functional evolutionary approach (7. ed.). Belmont, Calif. [u.a.]: Thomson, Brooks/Cole. ISBN 0-03-025982-7
- Applegate, Edith; Kent Van De Graaff. "The Skeletal System". Archived from the original on 2010-06-03. Retrieved 2009-01-03
- Bergmann O, Bhardwaj RD, Bernard S, et al. (April 2009). "Evidence for cardiomyocyte renewal in humans". Science. 324 (5923): 98–102. PMC 2991140. PMID 19342590. doi:10.1126/science.1164680
- Wickstead B, Gull K (Aug 2011). "The evolution of the cytoskeleton". The Journal of Cell Biology. 194 (4): 513–25. PMC 3160578. PMID 21859859. doi:10.1083/jcb.201102065
- Hardin, Jeff; Bertoni, Gregory; Kleinsmith, Lewis J. (2015). Becker's World of the Cell (8th ed.). New York: Pearson. pp. 422–446. ISBN 978013399939-6
- Rocca, Julius (9 August 2010). "A Note on Marinus of Alexandria". Journal of the History of the Neurosciences. 11 (3): 282–285. doi:10.1076/jhin.11.3.282.10386

- MacIntosh, BR; Gardiner, PF; McComas, AJ (2006). "1. Muscle Architecture and Muscle Fiber Anatomy". Skeletal Muscle: Form and Function (2nd ed.). Champaign, IL: Human Kinetics. pp. 3–21. ISBN 0-7360-4517-1
- Colliander EB, Tesch PA (1990). "Effects of eccentric and concentric muscle actions in resistance training". Acta Physiol. Scand. 140 (1): 31–9. PMID 2275403. doi:10.1111/j.1748-1716.1990.tb08973.x
- "Neurologic". The American Heritage Dictionary of the English Language, Fourth Edition. Houghton Mifflin Company. 2006. Retrieved 2008-11-15
- Roche, Alex F. (1994). "Sarcopenia: A critical review of its measurements and health-related significance in the middle-aged and elderly". American Journal of Human Biology. 6: 33–42. doi:10.1002/ajhb.1310060107
- Pedersen, B. K. (2013). "Muscle as a Secretory Organ". Comprehensive Physiology. Comprehensive Physiology. 3. pp. 1337–62. ISBN 9780470650714. PMID 23897689. doi:10.1002/cphy.c120033
- Ker, R. F., (2002). "The implications of the adaptable fatigue quality of tendons for their construction, repair and function". Comparative Biochemistry and Physiology A. 133 (4): 987–1000. PMID 12485688. doi:10.1016/S1095-6433(02)00171-X
- Fabiato, A. (1983). "Calcium-induced calcium release from the cardiac sarcoplasmic reticulum". American Journal of Physiology. 245 (1): C1–14. PMID 6346892
- Saladin, Kenneth (2012). Anatomy and Physiology: The Unity of Form and Function. New York: McGraw Hill. ISBN 978-0-07-337825-1
- Mackenzie, Colin (1918). The Action of Muscles: Including Muscle Rest and Muscle Re-education. England: Paul B. Hoeber. p. 1. Retrieved 18 April 2015
- Organ, Chris L. (2006). "Biomechanics of ossified tendons in ornithopod dinosaurs". Paleobiology. 32 (4): 652–665. doi:10.1666/05039.1

3

An Overview of Locomotion

One of the methods of human locomotion is crawling. The types of crawls are bear crawl, bridge walk, standard crawl, leopard crawl, tiger crawl, etc. Walking and running, trotting, etc. are other forms of human locomotion. This chapter is an overview of the subject matter incorporating all the major aspects of biomechanics.

Crawling (Human)

Crawling or Quadrupedal movement is a method of human locomotion that makes use of all four limbs. It is one of the earliest gaits learned by human infants, and has similar features to four-limbed movement in other primates and in non-primate quadrupeds.

When Crawls are used

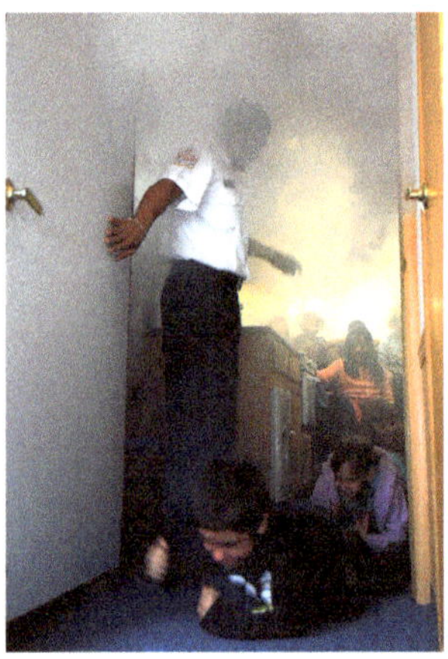

Children crawling on the ground during a fire drill in Italy.

Crawling is used mainly:

- When a person cannot yet walk because of being an infant
- When a person cannot walk due to disability, being wounded, sick, or drunk
- In very low places (caves, under a table, in a mine, etc.). Sometimes underground miners need to crawl long distances during their work
- When searching for something on the ground

- To get down to the ground in gardening, for maintenance or other work-related purposes which require a good reach on the ground
- For stealth (camouflage and quietness)
- To lower the field of vision
- As an exercise
- As a token of submission
- For fun or comical purposes
- During a fire, crawling may be used because the air near the ground is easier to breathe

In Infants

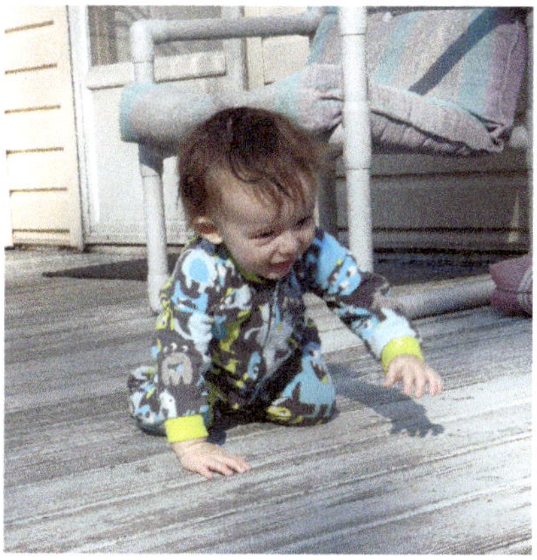

A 10-month-old baby crawling by kneeling.

Infants sometimes "crawl" with their stomachs on the ground as early as 3 months, but this crawling is infrequent with the baby remaining stationary most of the time. True crawling with the stomach off the ground and the baby frequently on the move usually develops between 7 and 11 months of age and lasts anywhere from a week to 4 months before the child switches to walking. Even after taking their first unaided steps, most babies still crawl part of the time until they have mastered walking. While crawling, infants gradually practice standing, at first by using people or objects for support and, later, without support. Crawling babies are notorious for getting into trouble, so parents are often advised to childproof their house before a baby reaches crawling age.

Though crawling is an important developmental milestone in children, it is not necessary for healthy development. Some babies skip crawling and go directly to walking. Others "bottom shuffle" instead of crawling (sometimes referred to as "bum-shuffling", or "scooting"). Bottom-shuffling babies sit on their bottoms and push themselves forward using their legs, and sometimes their hands, often in specially reinforced trousers. Babies that bottom-shuffle tend to walk later than babies that crawl.

Whether infants crawl is also culturally determined. European parents in previous centuries discouraged it as being too animal-like. They kept their children in long dresses and other clothes that made crawling difficult or impossible. Some cultures consider it to be dirty and dangerous.

Types of Crawls

Standard Crawl

Crawling is a specific 4-beat gait involving the hands and knees. A typical crawl is left-hand, right-knee, right-hand, left-knee, or a hand, the diagonal knee, the other hand then its diagonal knee. This is the first gait most humans learn, and is mainly used during early childhood, or when looking for something on the floor or under low relief. It can be used to move with a lower silhouette, but there are better crawls for that purpose. This is the most natural of the crawls and is the one that requires the least effort.

Bear Crawl

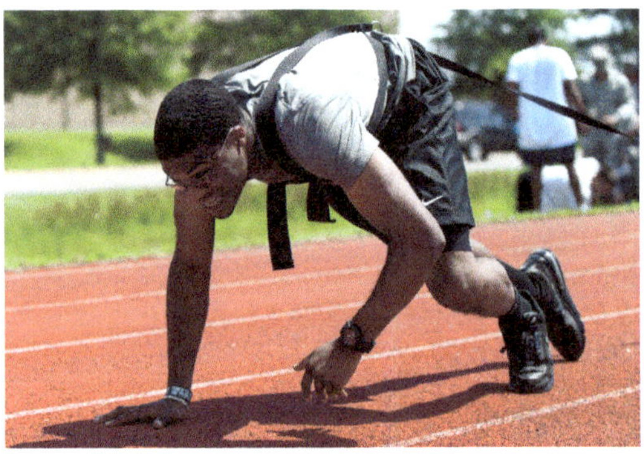

US Airman performs a bear crawl

The bear crawl is almost identical to the standard crawl, but the feet are used instead of the knees, which creates an arched or squatted body posture. This works as a faster crawl but requires more effort to maintain.

Bridge Walk

This involves holding a gymnastic bridge and making small steps with the arms and legs. It is similar to a crab walk in that the body locomotes in a supine posture, but the arms are in shoulder flexion alongside the head.

Because of its unusual appearance, crabwalking has been used in several horror films to suggest the demonic possession of a character. These have included *The Exorcist* and *The Unborn*. Wrestler Bray Wyatt does this.

Crab Crawl

The crab crawl is used in crab soccer. It starts by sitting down with the feet and hands flat on the ground, the hips are then raised off the ground and the chest faces the sky. It is similar to a bridge walk in that both have quadripedal locomotion with a supine torso, but here the arms are held behind the torso, with the shoulder joint being in hyperextension. Due to its inefficiency, it is more commonly used as a form of exercise than actual transportation. Crabwalking builds triceps endurance and arm and leg strength, and is a recommended exercise of various school athletic departments and soccer organizations, such as USA football.

The crab crawl is also useful for descending steep slopes with poor traction. Its feet-first orientation ensures a low center of mass to prevent tumbling, while the inverted posture allows one to see where they're going.

Leopard Crawl/High Crawl

Soldier crawls through mud during training

The leopard crawl is a military-specific crawl. There are two versions, the leopard crawl proper and a modified version for when carrying weapons in the hands. This is a two-beat gait like a trot: an arm/elbow is advanced with the diagonal knee. This is designed for the smallest silhouette possible, and the body is often nearly or actually touching the ground, and although the elbow and knee are the main focus, most of the respective limbs touch the ground.

Tiger Crawl

The tiger crawl is essentially a highly accelerated combination between crawl and leopard crawl. It uses the hands and the knees/feet depending upon the situation, while maintaining a silhouette almost as small as that of the leopard crawl. This is relatively fast gait but can take large amounts of energy.

Walking

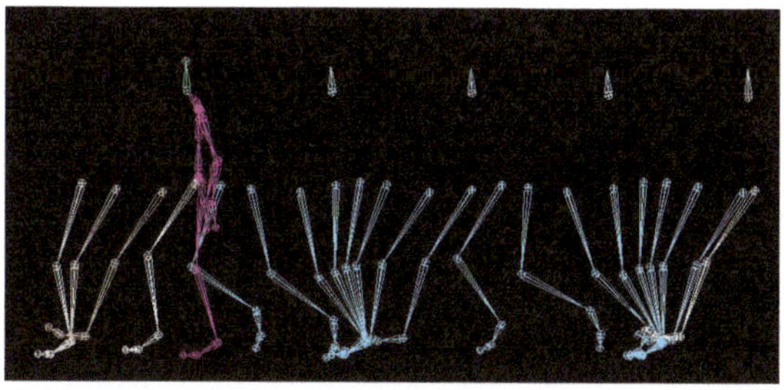

Computer simulation of a human walk cycle. In this model the head keeps the same level at all times, whereas the hip follows a sine curve.

Walking (also known as ambulation) is one of the main gaits of locomotion among legged animals. Walking is typically slower than running and other gaits. Walking is defined by an 'inverted pendulum' gait in which the body vaults over the stiff limb or limbs with each step. This applies regardless of the number of limbs - even arthropods, with six, eight or more limbs, walk.

Difference from Running

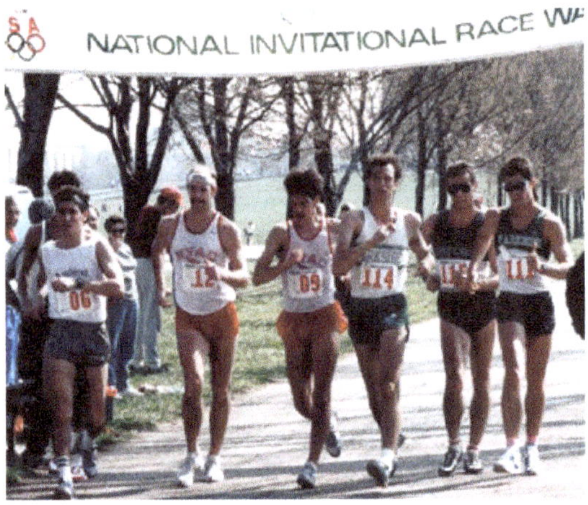

Racewalkers at the World Cup Trials in 1987

The word *walk* is descended from the Old English *wealcan* "to roll". In humans and other bipeds, walking is generally distinguished from running in that only one foot at a time leaves contact with the ground and there is a period of double-support. In contrast, running begins when both feet are off the ground with each step. This distinction has the status of a formal requirement in competitive walking events. For quadrupedal species, there are numerous gaits which may be termed walking or running, and distinctions based upon the presence or absence of a suspended phase or the number of feet in contact any time do not yield mechanically correct classification. The most effective method to distinguish walking from running is to measure the height of a person's centre of mass using motion capture or a force plate at midstance. During walking, the centre of mass reaches a maximum height at midstance, while during running, it is then at a minimum. This distinction, however, only holds true for locomotion over level or approximately level ground. For walking up grades above 9%, this distinction no longer holds for some individuals. Definitions based on the percentage of the stride during which a foot is in contact with the ground (averaged across all feet) of greater than 50% contact corresponds well with identification of 'inverted pendulum' mechanics and are indicative of walking for animals with any number of limbs, although this definition is incomplete. Running humans and animals may have contact periods greater than 50% of a gait cycle when rounding corners, running uphill or carrying loads.

Speed is another factor that distinguishes walking from running. Although walking speeds can vary greatly depending on many factors such as height, weight, age, terrain, surface, load, culture, effort, and fitness, the average human walking speed is about 5.0 kilometres per hour (km/h), or about 3.1 miles per hour (mph). Specific studies have found pedestrian walking speeds ranging from 4.51 kilometres per hour (2.80 mph) to 4.75 kilometres per hour (2.95 mph) for older individuals and from 5.32 kilometres per hour (3.31 mph) to 5.43 kilometres per hour (3.37 mph) for younger individuals; a brisk walking speed can be around 6.5 kilometres per hour (4.0 mph). Champion racewalkers can average more than 14 kilometres per hour (8.7 mph) over a distance of 20 kilometres (12 mi).

An average human child achieves independent walking ability at around 11 months old.

Health Benefits

Regular, brisk exercise of any kind can improve confidence, stamina, energy, weight control and life expectancy and reduce stress. It can also reduce the risk of coronary heart disease, strokes, diabetes, high blood pressure, bowel cancer and osteoporosis. Scientific studies have also shown that walking, besides its physical benefits, is also beneficial for the mind, improving memory skills, learning ability, concentration and abstract reasoning, as well as ameliorating spirits. Sustained walking sessions for a minimum period of thirty to sixty minutes a day, five days a week, with the correct walking posture, reduce health risks and have various overall health benefits, such as reducing the chances of cancer, type 2 diabetes, heart disease, anxiety disorder and depression. Life expectancy is also increased even for individuals suffering from obesity or high blood pressure. Walking also improves bone health, especially strengthening the hip bone, and lowering the harmful low-density lipoprotein (LDL) cholesterol, and raising the useful high-density lipoprotein (HDL) cholesterol. Studies have found that walking may also help prevent dementia and Alzheimer's.

The Centers for Disease Control and Prevention's fact sheet on the "Relationship of Walking to Mortality Among U.S. Adults with Diabetes" states that those with diabetes who walked for 2 or more hours a week lowered their mortality rate from all causes by 39 per cent. "Walking lengthened the life of people with diabetes regardless of age, sex, race, body mass index, length of time since diagnosis, and presence of complications or functional limitations." It has been suggested that there is a relationship between the speed of walking and health, and that the best results are obtained with a speed of more than 2.5 mph (4 km/h).

Governments now recognize the benefits of walking for mental and physical health and are actively encouraging it. This growing emphasis on walking has arisen because people walk less nowadays than previously. In the UK, a Department of Transport report found that between 1995/97 and 2005 the average number of walk trips per person fell by 16%, from 292 to 245 per year. Many professionals in local authorities and the NHS are employed to halt this decline by ensuring that the built environment allows people to walk and that there are walking opportunities available to them. Professionals working to encourage walking come mainly from six sectors: health, transport, environment, schools, sport and recreation, and urban design.

One programme to encourage walking is "The Walking the Way to Health Initiative", organized by the British walkers association The Ramblers, which is the largest volunteer led walking scheme in the United Kingdom. Volunteers are trained to lead free Health Walks from community venues such as libraries and doctors' surgeries. The scheme has trained over 35,000 volunteers and have over 500 schemes operating across the UK, with thousands of people walking every week. A new organization called "Walk England" launched a web site in June 2008 to provide these professionals with evidence, advice and examples of success stories of how to encourage communities to walk more. The site has a social networking aspect to allow professionals and the public to ask questions, post news and events and communicate with others in their area about walking, as well as a "walk now" option to find out what walks are available in each region. Similar organizations exist in other countries and recently a "Walking Summit" was held in the United States. This "assembl[ed] thought-leaders and influencers from business, urban planning and real estate, [along with] physicians and public health officials," and others, to discuss how to make American cities and communities places where "people can and want to walk".

It is theorized that "walking" among tetrapods originated underwater with air-breathing fish that could "walk" underwater, giving rise to the plethora of land-dwelling life that walk on four or two limbs. While terrestrial tetrapods are theorised to have a single origin, arthropods and their relatives are thought to have independently evolved walking several times, specifically in insects, myriapods, chelicerates, tardigrades, onychophorans, and crustaceans.

Judging from footprints discovered on a former shore in Kenya, it is thought possible that ancestors of modern humans were walking in ways very similar to the present activity as many as 1.5 million years ago.

Variants

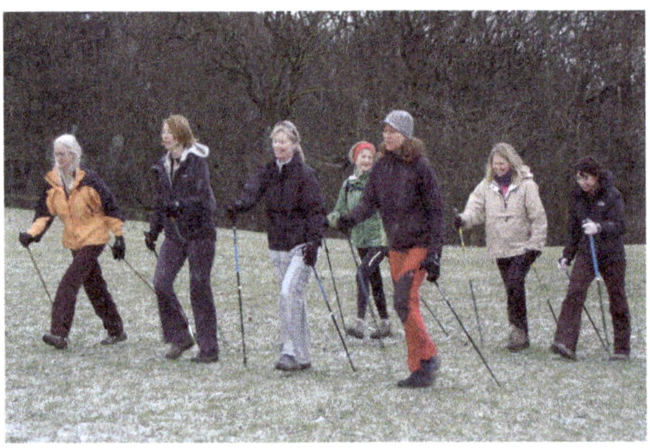

Nordic walkers

- Scrambling is a method of ascending a hill or mountain that involves using both hands, because of the steepness of the terrain. Of necessity it will be a slow and careful form of walking and with possibly of occasional brief, easy rock climbing. Some scrambling takes place on narrow exposed ridges where more attention to balance will be required than in normal walking.

- Snow shoeing—A snowshoe is footwear for walking over the snow. Snowshoes work by distributing the weight of the person over a larger area so that the person's foot does not sink completely into the snow, a quality called "flotation". It is often said by snowshoers that if you can walk, you can snowshoe. This is true in optimal conditions, but snowshoeing properly requires some slight adjustments to walking. The method of walking is to lift the shoes slightly and slide the inner edges over each other, thus avoiding the unnatural and fatiguing "straddle-gait" that would otherwise be necessary. A snowshoer must be willing to roll his or her feet slightly as well. An exaggerated stride works best when starting out, particularly with larger or traditional shoes.

- Beach walking is a sport that is based on walk on the sand of the beach. Beach walking can be developed on compact sand or non-compact sand. There are beach walking competitions on non-compact sand. And there are world records of beach walking on non-compact sand in Multiday distances. Beach walking has a specific technique of walk.

- Nordic walking is a physical activity and a sport, which is performed with specially designed walking poles similar to ski poles. Compared to regular walking, Nordic walking (also called pole walking) involves applying force to the poles with each stride. Nordic walkers use more of their entire body (with greater intensity) and receive fitness building stimulation not present in normal walking for the chest, lats, triceps, biceps, shoulder, abdominals, spinal and other core muscles that may result in significant increases in heart rate at a given pace. Nordic walking has been estimated as producing up to a 46% increase in energy consumption, compared to walking without poles.

- Pedestrianism is a sport that developed during the late eighteenth and nineteenth centuries, and was a popular spectator sport in the British Isles. By the end of the 18th century, and especially with the growth of the popular press, feats of foot travel over great distances (similar to a modern ultramarathon) gained attention, and were labeled "pedestrianism". Interest in the sport, and the wagering which accompanied it, spread to the United States, Canada, and Australia in the 19th century. By the end of the 19th century, Pedestrianism was largely displaced by the rise in modern spectator sports and by controversy involving rules, which limited its appeal as a source of wagering and led to its inclusion in the amateur athletics movement. Pedestrianism was first codified in the last half of the 19th century, evolving into what would become racewalking, By the mid 19th century, competitors were often expected to extend their legs straight at least once in their stride, and obey what was called the "fair heel and toe" rule. This rule, the source of modern racewalking, was a vague commandment that the toe of one foot could not leave the ground before the heel of the next foot touched down. This said, rules were customary and changed with competition. Racers were usually allowed to jog in order to fend off cramps, and it was distance, not code, which determined gait for longer races. Newspaper reports suggest that "trotting" was common in events.

- Power walking or speed walking is the act of walking with a speed at the upper end of the natural range for walking gait, typically 7 to 9 km/h (4.5 to 5.5 mph). To qualify as power walking as opposed to jogging or running, at least one foot must be in contact with the ground at all times.
- Racewalking is a long-distance athletic event. Although it is a foot race, it is different from running in that one foot must appear to be in contact with the ground at all times. Stride length is reduced, so to achieve competitive speeds, racewalkers must attain cadence rates comparable to those achieved by Olympic 800-meter runners, and they must do so for hours at a time since the Olympic events are the 20 km (12.4 mi) race walk (men and women) and 50 km (31 mi) race walk (men only), and 50 mile (80.5 km) events are also held.
- Afghan walking: The Afghan Walk is a rhythmic breathing technique synchronized with walking. It was born in the 1980s on the basis of the observations made by the Frenchman Édouard G. Stiegler, during his contacts with Afghan caravaners, capable of making walks of more than 60 km per day for dozens of days.

Biomechanics

Human walking is accomplished with a strategy called the double pendulum. During forward motion, the leg that leaves the ground swings forward from the hip. This sweep is the first pendulum. Then the leg strikes the ground with the heel and rolls through to the toe in a motion described as an inverted pendulum. The motion of the two legs is coordinated so that one foot or the other is always in contact with the ground. The process of walking recovers approximately sixty per cent of the energy used due to pendulum dynamics and ground reaction force.

Walking differs from a running gait in a number of ways. The most obvious is that during walking one leg always stays on the ground while the other is swinging. In running there is typically a ballistic phase where the runner is airborne with both feet in the air (for bipedals).

Another difference concerns the movement of the centre of mass of the body. In walking the body "vaults" over the leg on the ground, raising the centre of mass to its highest point as the leg passes the vertical, and dropping it to the lowest as the legs are spread apart. Essentially kinetic energy of forward motion is constantly being traded for a rise in potential energy. This is reversed in running where the centre of mass is at its lowest as the leg is vertical. This is because the impact of landing from the ballistic phase is absorbed by bending the leg and consequently storing energy in muscles and tendons. In running there is a conversion between kinetic, potential, and elastic energy.

There is an absolute limit on an individual's speed of walking (without special techniques such as those employed in speed walking) due to the upwards acceleration of the centre of mass during a stride - if it's greater than the acceleration due to gravity the person will become airborne as they vault over the leg on the ground. Typically however, animals switch to a run at a lower speed than this due to energy efficiencies.

A Leisure Activity

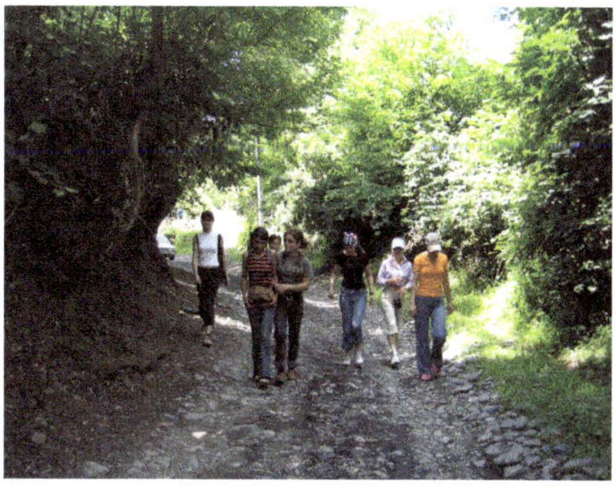

Walking in Shilda, Georgia

Many people enjoy walking as a recreation in the mainly urban modern world, and it is one of the best forms of exercise. For some, walking is a way to enjoy nature and the outdoors; and for others the physical, sporting and endurance aspect is more important.

There are a variety of different kinds of walking, including bushwalking, racewalking, beach walking, hillwalking, volksmarching, Nordic walking, trekking and hiking. Some people prefer to walk indoors on a treadmill, or in a gym, and fitness walkers and others may use a pedometer to count their steps. Hiking is the usual word used in Canada, the United States and South Africa for long vigorous walks; similar walks are called tramps in New Zealand, or hill walking or just walking in Australia, the UK and the Irish Republic. Australians also bushwalk. In English-speaking parts of North America the term walking is used for short walks, especially in towns and cities. Snow shoeing is walking in snow; a slightly different gait is required compared with regular walking.

In terms of tourism the possibilities range from guided walking tours in cities, to organized trekking holidays in the Himalayas. In the UK the term walking tour also refers to a multi-day walk or hike undertaken by a group or individual. Well-organized systems of trails exist in many other European counties, as well as Canada, United States, New Zealand, and Nepal. Systems of lengthy waymarked walking trails now stretch across Europe from Norway to Turkey, Portugal to Cyprus. Many also walk the traditional pilgrim routes, of which the most famous is El Camino de Santiago, The Way of St. James.

Numerous walking festivals and other walking events take place each year in many countries. The world's largest multi-day walking event is the International Four Days Marches Nijmegen in the Netherlands. The "Vierdaagse" (Dutch for "Four day Event") is an annual walk that has taken place since 1909; it has been based at Nijmegen since 1916. Depending on age group and category, walkers have to walk 30, 40 or 50 kilometers each day for four days. Originally a military event with a few civilians, it now is a mainly civilian event. Numbers have risen in recent years, with over 40,000 now taking part, including about 5,000 military personnel. Due to crowds on the route, since 2004 the organizers have limited the number of participants. In the U.S., there is the annual Labor Day walk on Mackinac Bridge, Michigan, which draws over 60,000 participants; it is the largest single-day walking event; while the Chesapeake Bay Bridge Walk in Maryland draws over 50,000 participants each year. There are also various walks organised as charity events, with walkers sponsored for a specific cause. Thes walks range in length from two miles (3 km) or five km to 50 miles (80 km). The MS Challenge Walk is an 80 km or 50 mile walk which raises money to fight multiple sclerosis, while walkers in the Oxfam Trailwalker cover 100 km or 60 miles.

In Britain, The Ramblers, a registered charity, is the largest organisation that looks after the interests of walkers, with some 139,000 members. Its "Get Walking Keep Walking" project provides free route guides, led walks, as well as information for people new to walking. The Long Distance Walkers Association in the UK is for the more energetic walker, and organizes lengthy challenge hikes of 20 or even 50 miles (30 to 80 km) or more in a day. The LDWA's annual "Hundred" event, entailing walking 100 miles or 160 km in 48 hours, takes place each British Spring Bank Holiday weekend.

Walkability

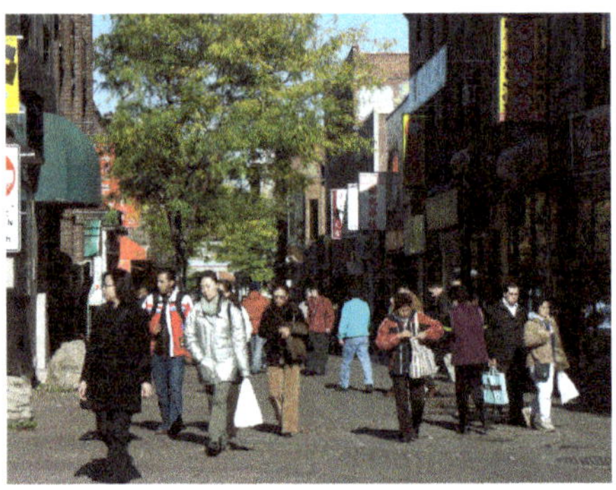

Gauchetière Street, Montreal, Canada

There has been a recent focus among urban planners in some communities to create pedestrian-friendly areas and roads, allowing commuting, shopping and recreation to be done on foot. The concept of walkability has arisen as a measure of the degree to which an area is friendly to walking. Some communities are at least partially car-free, making them particularly supportive of walking and other modes of transportation. In the United States, the active living network is an example of a concerted effort to develop communities more friendly to walking and other physical activities.

An example of such efforts to make urban development more pedestrian friendly is the pedestrian village. This is a compact, pedestrian-oriented neighborhood or town, with a mixed-use village center, that follows the tenets of New Pedestrianism. Shared-use lanes for pedestrians and those using bicycles, Segways, wheelchairs, and other small rolling conveyances that do not use internal combustion engines. Generally, these lanes are in front of the houses and businesses, and streets for motor vehicles are always at the rear. Some pedestrian villages might be nearly car-free with cars either hidden below the buildings or on the periphery of the village. Venice, Italy is essentially a pedestrian village with canals. The canal district in Venice, California, on the other hand, combines the front lane/rear street approach with canals and walkways, or just walkways.

Walking is also considered to be a clear example of a sustainable mode of transport, especially suited for urban use and/or relatively shorter distances. Non-motorised transport modes such as walking, but also cycling, small-wheeled transport (skates, skateboards, push scooters and hand carts) or wheelchair travel are often key elements of successfully encouraging clean urban transport. A large variety of case studies and good practices (from European cities and some worldwide examples) that promote and stimulate walking as a means of transportation in cities can be found at Eltis, Europe's portal for local transport.

The development of specific rights of way with appropriate infrastructure can promote increased participation and enjoyment of walking. Examples of types of investment include pedestrian malls, and foreshoreways such as oceanways and also river walks.

The first purpose-built pedestrian street in Europe is the Lijnbaan in Rotterdam, opened in 1953. The first pedestrianised shopping centre in the United Kingdom was in Stevenage in 1959. A large number of European towns and cities have made part of their centres car-free since the early 1960s. These are often accompanied by car parks on the edge of the pedestrianised zone, and, in the larger cases, park and ride schemes. Central Copenhagen is one of the largest and oldest: It was converted from car traffic into pedestrian zone in 1962.

In Robotics

The first successful attempts at walking robots tended to have six legs. The number of legs was reduced as microprocessor technology advanced, and there are now a number of robots that can walk on two legs. One, for example, is ASIMO. Although robots have taken great strides in advancement, they still don't walk nearly as well as human beings as they often need to keep their knees bent permanently in order to improve stability.

In 2009, Japanese roboticist Tomotaka Takahashi developed a robot that can jump three inches off the ground. The robot, named Ropid, is capable of getting up, walking, running, and jumping.

Animals

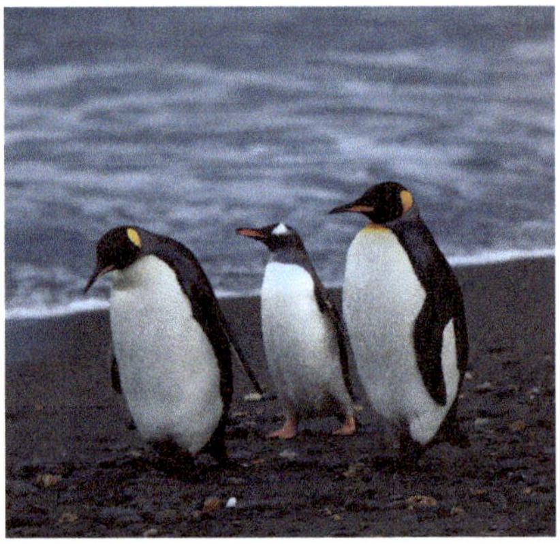

Two king penguins and one gentoo penguin walking on a beach on South Georgia, British overseas territory.

Horses

The walk is a four-beat gait that averages about 4 miles per hour (6.4 km/h). When walking, a horse's legs follow this sequence: left hind leg, left front leg, right hind leg, right front leg, in a regular 1-2-3-4 beat. At the walk, the horse will always have one foot raised and the other three feet on the ground, save for a brief moment when weight is being transferred from one foot to another. A horse moves its head and neck in a slight up and down motion that helps maintain balance.

Ideally, the advancing rear hoof oversteps the spot where the previously advancing front hoof touched the ground. The more the rear hoof oversteps, the smoother and more comfortable the walk becomes. Individual horses and different breeds vary in the smoothness of their walk. However, a rider will almost always feel some degree of gentle side-to-side motion in the horse's hips as each hind leg reaches forward.

The fastest "walks" with a four-beat footfall pattern are actually the lateral forms of ambling gaits such as the running walk, singlefoot, and similar rapid but smooth intermediate speed gaits. If a horse begins to speed up and lose a regular four-beat cadence to its gait, the horse is no longer walking, but is beginning to either trot or pace.

Elephants

Elephants can move both forwards and backwards, but cannot trot, jump, or gallop. They use only two gaits when moving on land, the walk and a faster gait similar to running. In walking, the legs act as pendulums, with the hips and shoulders rising and falling while the foot is planted on the ground. With no "aerial phase", the fast gait does not meet all the criteria of running, although the elephant uses its legs much like other running animals, with the hips and shoulders falling and then rising while the feet are on the ground. Fast-moving elephants appear to 'run' with their front legs, but 'walk' with their hind legs and can reach a top speed of 18 km/h (11 mph). At this speed, most other quadrupeds are well into a gallop, even accounting for leg length.

Walking Fish

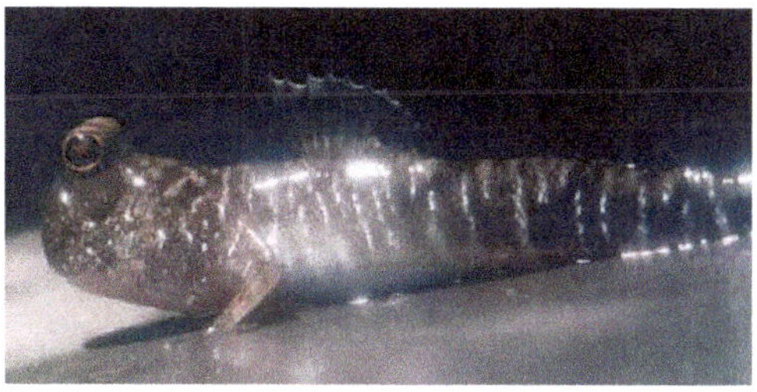

A mudskipper, a type of walking fish, perched on land.

Walking fish, sometimes called ambulatory fish, is a general term that refers to fish that are able to travel over land for extended periods of time. The term may also be used for some other cases of nonstandard fish locomotion, e.g., when describing fish "walking" along the sea floor, as the handfish or frogfish.

Running

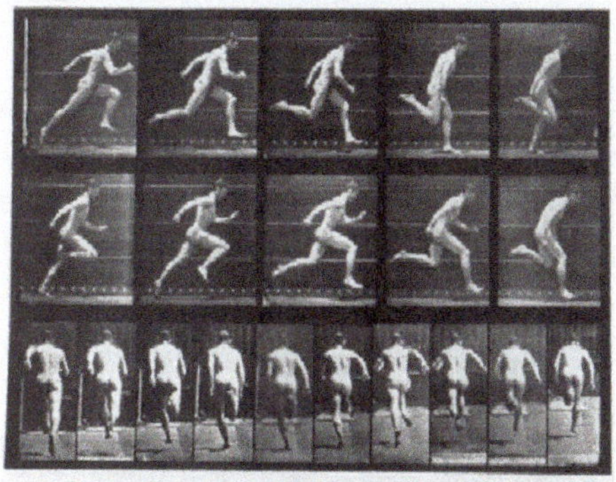

Eadweard Muybridge photo sequence

Running is a method of terrestrial locomotion allowing humans and other animals to move rapidly on foot. Running is a type of gait characterized by an aerial phase in which all feet are above the ground (though there are exceptions). This is in contrast to walking, where one foot is always in contact with the ground, the legs are kept mostly straight and the center of gravity vaults over the stance leg or legs in an inverted pendulum fashion. A characteristic feature of a running body from the viewpoint of spring-mass mechanics is that changes in kinetic and potential energy within a stride occur simultaneously, with energy storage accomplished by springy tendons and passive muscle elasticity. The term running can refer to any of a variety of speeds ranging from jogging to sprinting.

It is assumed that the ancestors of mankind developed the ability to run for long distances about 2.6 million years ago, probably in order to hunt animals. Competitive running grew out of religious festivals in various areas. Records of competitive racing date back to the Tailteann Games in Ireland in 1829 BCE, while the first recorded Olympic Games took place in 776 BCE. Running has been described as the world's most accessible sport.

History

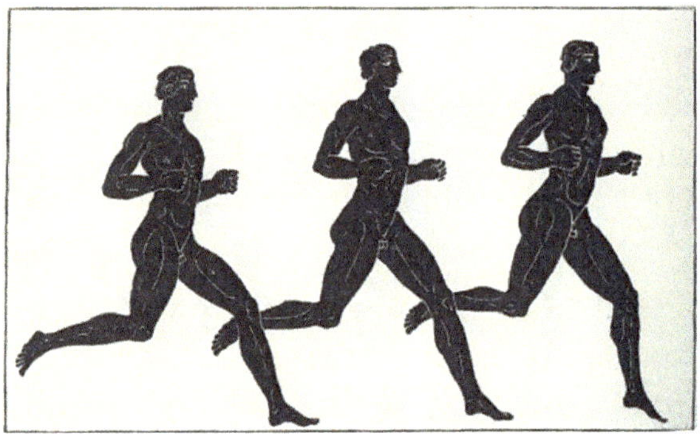

A scene depicting long distance runners, originally found on a Panathenaic amphora from Ancient Greece, circa 333 B.C.

It is thought that human running evolved at least four and a half million years ago out of the ability of the ape-like Australopithecus, an early ancestor of humans, to walk upright on two legs.

The theory proposed considered to be the most likely evolution of running is of early humans' developing as endurance runners from the practice of persistence hunting of animals, the activity of following and chasing until a prey is too exhausted to flee, succumbing to "chase myopathy" (Sears 2001), and that human features such as the nuchal ligament, abundant sweat glands, the Achilles tendons, big knee joints and muscular glutei maximi, were changes caused by this type of activity (Bramble & Lieberman 2004, et al.). The theory as first proposed used comparative physiological evidence and the natural habits of animals when running, indicating the likelihood of this activity as a successful hunting method. Further evidence from observation of modern-day hunting practice also indicated this likelihood (Carrier et al. 1984). According to Sears (p. 12) scientific investigation (Walker & Leakey 1993) of the Nariokotome Skeleton provided further evidence for the Carrier theory.

Competitive running grew out of religious festivals in various areas such as Greece, Egypt, Asia, and the East African Rift in Africa. The Tailteann Games, an Irish sporting festival in honor of the goddess Tailtiu, dates back to 1829 BCE, and is one of the earliest records of competitive running. The origins of the Olympics and Marathon running are shrouded by myth and legend, though the first recorded games took place in 776 BCE. Running in Ancient Greece can be traced back to these games of 776 BCE.

...I suspect that the sun, moon, earth, stars, and heaven, which are still the Gods of many barbarians, were the only Gods known to the aboriginal Hellenes. Seeing that they were always moving and running, from their running nature they were called Gods or runners (Thus, Theontas)...

—*Socrates in Plato - Cratylus*

Running Kinematic Description

Running gait can be divided into two phases in regard to the lower extremity: stance and swing. These can be further divided into absorption, propulsion, initial swing and terminal swing. Due to the continuous nature of running gait, no certain point is assumed to be the beginning. However, for simplicity it will be assumed that absorption and footstrike mark the beginning of the running cycle in a body already in motion.

Footstrike

Footstrike occurs when a plantar portion of the foot makes initial contact with the ground. Common footstrike types include forefoot, midfoot and heel strike types. These are characterized by initial contact of the ball of the foot, ball and heel of the foot simultaneously and heel of the foot respectively. During this time the hip joint is undergoing extension from being in maximal flexion from the previous swing phase. For proper force absorption, the knee joint should be flexed upon footstrike and the ankle should be slightly in front of the body. Footstrike begins the absorption phase as forces from initial contact are attenuated throughout the lower extremity. Absorption of forces continues as the body moves from footstrike to midstance due to vertical propulsion from the toe-off during a previous gait cycle.

Midstance

Midstance is defined as the time at which the lower extremity limb of focus is in knee flexion directly underneath the trunk, pelvis and hips. It is at this point that propulsion begins to occur as the hips undergo hip extension, the knee joint undergoes extension and the ankle undergoes plantar flexion. Propulsion continues until the leg is extended behind the body and toe off occurs. This involves maximal hip extension, knee extension and plantar flexion for the subject, resulting in the body being pushed forward from this motion and the ankle/foot leaves the ground as initial swing begins.

Propulsion Phase

Most recent research, particularly regarding the footstrike debate, has focused solely on the absorption phases for injury identification and prevention purposes. The propulsion phase of running involves the movement beginning at midstance until toe off. From a full stride length model however, components of the terminal swing and footstrike can aid in propulsion. Set up for propulsion begins at the end of terminal swing as the hip joint flexes, creating the maximal range of motion for the hip extensors to accelerate through and produce force. As the hip extensors change from reciporatory inhibitors to primary muscle movers, the lower extremity is brought back toward the ground, although aided greatly by the stretch reflex and gravity. Footstrike and absorption phases occur next with two types of outcomes. This phase can be only a continuation of momentum from the stretch reflex reaction to hip flexion, gravity and light hip extension with a heel strike, which does little to provide force absorption through the ankle joint. With a mid/forefoot strike, loading of the gastro-soleus complex from shock absorption will serve to aid in plantar flexion from midstance to toe-off. As the lower extremity enters midstance, true propulsion begins. The hip extensors continue contracting along with help from the acceleration of gravity and the stretch reflex left over from maximal hip flexion during the terminal swing phase. Hip extension pulls the ground underneath the body, thereby pulling the runner forward. During midstance, the knee should be in some degree of knee flexion due to elastic loading from the absorption and footstrike phases to preserve forward momentum. The ankle joint is in dorsiflexion at this point underneath the body, either elastically loaded from a mid/forefoot strike or preparing for stand-alone concentric plantar flexion. All three joints perform the final propulsive movements during toe-off. The plantar flexors plantar flex, pushing off from the ground and returning from dorsiflexion in midstance. This can either occur by releasing the elastic load from an earlier mid/forefoot strike or concentrically contracting from a heel strike. With a forefoot strike, both the ankle and knee joints will release their stored elastic energy from the footstrike/absorption phase. The quadriceps group/knee extensors go into full knee extension, pushing the body off of the ground. At the same time, the knee flexors and stretch reflex pull the knee back into flexion, adding to a pulling motion on the ground and beginning the initial swing phase. The hip extensors extend to maximum, adding the forces pulling and pushing off of the ground. The movement and momentum generated by the hip extensors also contributes to knee flexion and the beginning of the initial swing phase.

Swing Phase

Initial swing is the response of both stretch reflexes and concentric movements to the propulsion movements of the body. Hip flexion and knee flexion occur beginning the return of the limb to the starting position and setting up for another footstrike. Initial swing ends at midswing, when the limb is again directly underneath the trunk, pelvis and hip with the knee joint flexed and hip flexion continuing. Terminal swing then begins as hip flexion continues to the point of activation of the stretch reflex of the hip extensors. The knee begins to extend slightly as it swings to the anterior portion of the body. The foot then makes contact with the ground with footstrike, completing the running cycle of one side of the lower extremity. Each limb of the lower extremity works opposite to the other. When one side is in toe-off/propulsion, the other hand is in the swing/recovery phase preparing for footstrike. Following toe-off and the beginning of the initial swing of one side, there is a flight phase where neither extremity is in contact with the ground due to the opposite side finishing terminal swing. As the footstrike of the one hand occurs, initial swing continues. The opposing limbs meet with one in mid-stance and midswing, beginning the propulsion and terminal swing phases.

Upper Extremity Function

Upper extremity function serves mainly in providing balance in conjunction with the opposing side of the lower extremity. The movement of each leg is paired with the opposite arm which serves to counterbalance the body, particularly during the stance phase. The arms move most effectively (as seen in elite athletes) with the elbow joint at an approximately 90 degrees or less, the hands swinging from the hips up to mid chest level with the opposite leg, the Humerus moving from being parallel with the trunk to approximately 45 degrees shoulder extension (never passing the trunk in flexion) and with as little movement in the transverse plane as possible. The trunk also rotates in conjunction with arm swing. It mainly serves as a balance point from which the limbs are anchored. Thus trunk motion should remain mostly stable with little motion except for slight rotation as excessive movement would contribute to transverse motion and wasted energy.

Footstrike Debate

Recent research into various forms of running has focused on the differences, in the potential injury risks and shock absorption capabilities between heel and mid/forefoot footstrikes. It has been shown that heel striking is generally associated with higher rates of injury and impact due to inefficient shock absorption and inefficient biomechanical compensations for these forces. This is due to forces from a heel strike traveling through bones for shock absorption rather than being absorbed by muscles. Since bones cannot disperse forces easily, the forces transmitted to other parts of the body, including ligaments, joints and bones in the rest of the lower extremity all the way up to the lower back. This causes the body to use abnormal compensatory motions in an attempt to avoid serious bone injuries. These compensations include internal rotation of the tibia, knee and hip joints. Excessive amounts of compensation over time have been linked to higher risk of injuries in those joints as well as the muscles involved in those motions. Conversely, a mid/forefoot strike has been associated with greater efficiency and lower injury risk due to the triceps surae being used as a lever system to absorb forces with the muscles eccentrically rather than through the bone. Landing with a mid/forefoot strike has also been shown to not only properly attenuate shock but allows the triceps surae to aid in propulsion via reflexive plantarflexion after stretching to absorb ground contact forces. Thus a mid/forefoot strike may aid in propulsion. However, even among elite athletes there are variations in self selected footstrike types. This is especially true in longer distance events, where there is a prevalence of heel strikers. There does tend however to be a greater percentage of mid/forefoot striking runners in the elite fields, particularly in the faster racers and the winning individuals or groups. While one could attribute the faster speeds of elite runners compared to recreational runners with similar footstrikes to physiological differences, the hip and joints have been left out of the equation for proper propulsion. This brings up the question as to how heel striking elite distance runners are able to keep up such high paces with a supposedly inefficient and injurious foot strike technique.

Stride Length, Hip and Knee Function

Biomechanical factors associated with elite runners include increased hip function, use and stride length over recreational runners. An increase in running speeds causes increased ground reaction forces and elite distance runners must compensate for this to maintain their pace over long distances. These forces are attenuated through increased stride length via increased hip flexion and extension through decreased ground contact time and more force being used in propulsion. With increased propulsion in the horizontal plane, less impact occurs from decreased force in the vertical plane. Increased hip flexion allows for increased use of the hip extensors through midstance and toe-off, allowing for more force production. The difference even between world class and national level distance runners has been associated with more efficient hip joint function. The increase in velocity likely comes from the increased range of motion in hip flexion and extension, allowing for greater acceleration and velocity. The hip extensors and hip extension have been linked to more powerful knee extension during toe-off, which contributes to propulsion. Stride length must be properly increased with some degree of knee flexion maintained through the terminal swing phases, as excessive knee extension during this phase along with footstrike has been associated with higher impact forces due to braking and an increased prevalence of heel striking. Elite runners tend to exhibit some degree of knee flexion at footstrike and midstance, which first serves to eccentrically absorb impact forces in the quadriceps muscle group. Secondly it allows for the knee joint to concentrically contract and provides major aid in propulsion during toe-off as the quadriceps group is capable of produce large amounts of force. Recreational runners have been shown to increase stride length through increased knee extension rather than increased hip flexion as exhibited by elite runners, which serves instead to provide an intense breaking motion with each step and decrease the rate and efficiency of knee extension during toe-off, slowing down speed. Knee extension however contributes to additional stride length and propulsion during toe-off and is seen more frequently in elite runners as well.

Elements of Good Running Technique

Upright Posture and a Slight Forward Lean

Leaning forward places a runner's center of mass on the front part of the foot, which avoids landing on the heel and facilitates the use of the spring mechanism of the foot. It also makes it easier for the runner to avoid landing the foot in front of the center of mass and the resultant braking effect. While upright posture is essential, a runner should maintain a relaxed frame and use his/her core to keep posture upright and stable. This helps prevent injury as long as the body is neither rigid nor tense. The most common running mistakes are tilting the chin up and scrunching shoulders.

Stride Rate and Types

Exercise physiologists have found that the stride rates are extremely consistent across professional runners, between 185 and 200 steps per minute. The main difference between long- and short-distance runners is the length of stride rather than the rate of stride.

During running, the speed at which the runner moves may be calculated by multiplying the cadence (steps per second) by the stride length. Running is often measured in terms of pace in minutes per mile or kilometer. Fast stride rates coincide with the rate one pumps one's arms. The faster one's arms move up and down, parallel with the body, the faster the rate of stride. Different types of stride are necessary for different types of running. When sprinting, runners stay on their toes bringing their legs up, using shorter and faster strides. Long distance runners tend to have more relaxed strides that vary.

Benefits of Running

Cardiovascular Benefits

While there exists the potential for injury while running (just as there is in any sport), there are many benefits. Some of these benefits include potential weight loss, improved cardiovascular and respiratory health (reducing the risk of cardiovascular and respiratory diseases), improved cardiovascular fitness, reduced total blood cholesterol, strengthening of bones (and potentially increased bone density), possible strengthening of the immune system and an improved self-esteem and emotional state. Running, like all forms of regular exercise, can effectively slow or reverse the effects of aging.

Whereby an optimal amount of vigorous aerobic exercise such as running might bring benefits related to lower cardiovascular disease and life extension, it should be noted that in an excessive dose (e.g., marathons) it might have an opposite effect associated with cardiotoxicity.

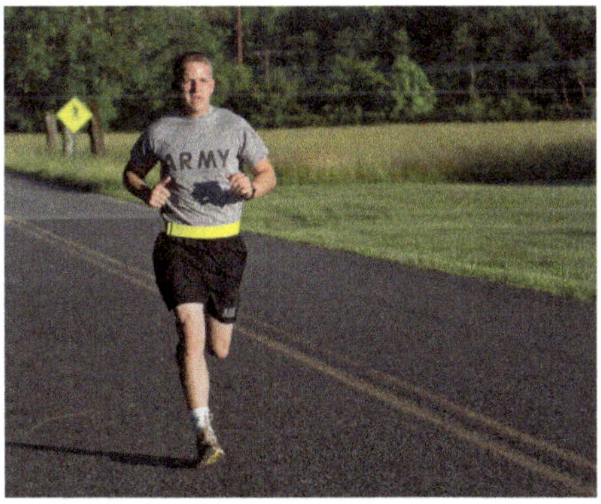

Soldier running to maintain his health

Weight Loss Benefits

Running can assist people in losing weight, staying in shape and improving body composition. Research suggests that for the person of average weight, they will burn approximately 100 calories per mile they run. Running increases your metabolism even after you have finished running. You will continue to burn an increased level of calories for a short time after the run. Different speeds and distances are appropriate for different individual health and fitness levels. For new runners, it takes time to get into shape. The key is consistency and a slow increase in speed and distance. While running, it is best to pay attention to how one's body feels. If a runner is gasping for breath or feels exhausted while running, it may be beneficial to slow down or try a shorter distance for a few weeks. If a runner feels that the pace or distance is no longer challenging, then the runner may want to speed up or run farther.

Mental Health

Running can also have psychological benefits, as many participants in the sport report feeling an elated, euphoric state, often referred to as a "runner's high". Running is frequently recommended as therapy for people with clinical depression and people coping with addiction. A possible benefit may be the enjoyment of nature and scenery, which also improves psychological well-being .

In animal models, running has been shown to increase the number of newly born neurons within the brain. This finding could have significant implications in aging as well as learning and memory. A recent study published in Cell Metabolism has also linked running with improved memory and learning skills.

Running Injuries

High Impact

Many injuries are associated with running because of its high-impact nature. Change in running volume may lead to development of patellofemoral pain syndrome, iliotibial band syndrome, patellar tendinopathy, plica syndrome, and medial tibial stress syndrome. Change in running pace may cause Achilles Tendinitis, gastrocnemius injuries, and plantar fasciitis. Repetitive stress on the same tissues without enough time for recovery or running with improper form can lead to many of the above. Runners generally attempt to minimize these injuries by warming up before exercise, focusing on proper running form, performing strength training exercises, eating a well balanced diet, allowing time for recovery, and "icing" (applying ice to sore muscles or taking an ice bath).

Some runners may experience injuries when running on concrete surfaces. The problem with running on concrete is that the body adjusts to this flat surface running, and some of the muscles will become weaker, along with the added impact of running on a harder surface. Therefore, it is advised to change terrain occasionally – such as trail, beach, or grass running. This is more unstable ground and allows the legs to strengthen different muscles. Runners should be wary of twisting their ankles on such terrain. Running downhill also increases knee stress and should, therefore, be avoided. Reducing the frequency and duration can also prevent injury.

Barefoot running has been promoted as a means of reducing running related injuries, but this remains controversial and a majority of professionals advocate the wearing of appropriate shoes as the best method for avoiding injury. However, a study in 2013 concluded that wearing neutral shoes is not associated with increased injuries.

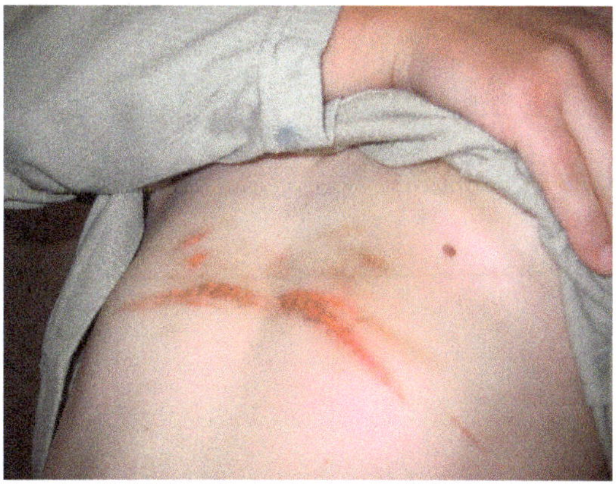

Chafing of skin following a marathon run

Chafing

Another common, running-related injury is chafing, caused by repetitive rubbing of one piece of skin against another, or against an article of clothing. One common location for chafe to occur is the runner's upper thighs. The skin feels coarse and develops a rash-like look. A variety of deodorants and special anti-chafing creams are available to treat such problems. Chafe is also likely to occur on the nipple. There are a variety of home remedies that runners use to deal with chafing while running such as band-aids and using grease to reduce friction. Prevention is key which is why form fitting cloths are important.

Running Events

Running is both a competition and a type of training for sports that have running or endurance components. As a sport, it is split into events divided by distance and sometimes includes permutations such as the obstacles in steeplechase and hurdles. Running races are contests to determine which of the competitors is able to run a certain distance in the shortest time. Today, competitive running events make up the core of the sport of athletics. Events are usually grouped into several classes, each requiring substantially different athletic strengths and involving different tactics, training methods, and types of competitors.

Running competitions have probably existed for most of humanity's history and were a key part of the ancient Olympic Games as well as the modern Olympics. The activity of running went through a period of widespread popularity in the United States during the running boom of the 1970s. Over the next two decades, as many as 25 million Americans were doing some form of running or jogging – accounting for roughly one tenth of the population. Today, road racing is a popular sport among non-professional athletes, who included over 7.7 million people in America alone in 2002.

Limits of Speed

Footspeed, or sprint speed, is the maximum speed at which a human can run. It is affected by many factors, varies greatly throughout the population, and is important in athletics and many sports.

The fastest human footspeed on record is 44.7 km/h (12.4 m/s, 27.8 mph), seen during a 100-meter sprint (average speed between the 60th and the 80th meter) by Usain Bolt.

Running Speed over Increasing Distance based on World Record Times

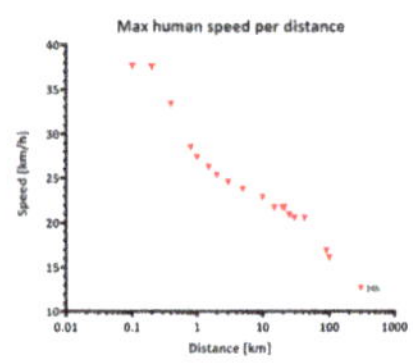

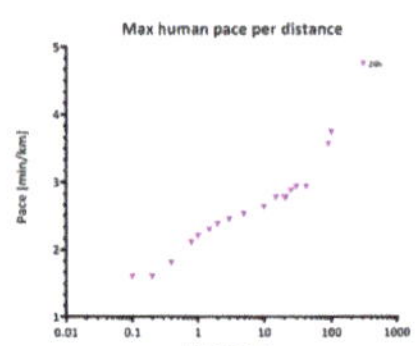

Maximum human speed [km/h] and pace [min/km] per distance (portrait orientation)

Distance metres	Men m/s	Women m/s
100	10.44	9.53
200	10.42	9.37
400	9.26	8.44
800	7.92	7.06
1,000	7.58	6.71
1,500	7.28	6.51
1,609 mile	7.22	6.36
2,000	7.02	6.15
3,000	6.81	6.17
5,000	6.60	5.87
10,000 track	6.34	5.64
10,000 road	6.23	5.49

15,000 road	6.02	5.38
20,000 track	5.91	5.09
20,000 road	6.02	5.30
21,097 Half marathon	6.02	5.29
21,285 One hour run	5.91	5.14
25,000 track	5.63	4.78
25,000 road	5.80	5.22
30,000 track	5.60	4.72
30,000 road	5.69	5.06
42,195 Marathon	5.69	5.19
90,000 Comrades	4.68	4.23
100,000	4.46	4.24
303,506 24-hour run	3.513	2.82

Events by Type

Track Running

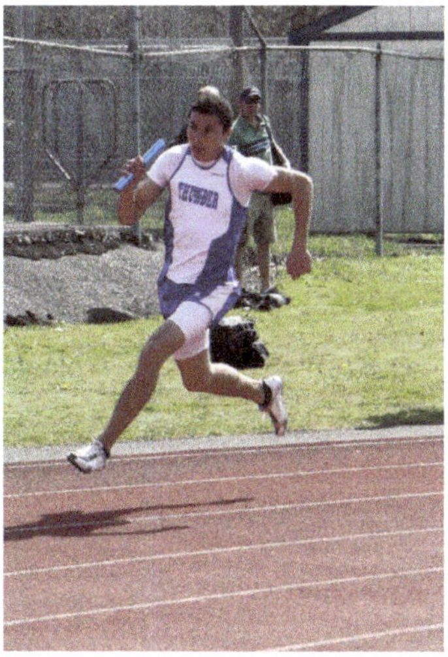

A man running with a baton during a relay race.

Track running events are individual or relay events with athletes racing over specified distances on an oval running track. The events are categorised as sprints, middle and long-distance, and hurdling.

Road Running

Road running takes place on a measured course over an established road (as opposed to track and cross country running). These events normally range from distances of 5 kilometers to longer distances such as half marathons and marathons, and they may involve scores of runners or wheelchair entrants.

Cross-country Running

Cross country running takes place over the open or rough terrain. The courses used for these events may include grass, mud, woodlands, hills, flat ground and water. It is a popular participatory sport and is one of the events which, along with track and field, road running, and racewalking, makes up the umbrella sport of athletics.

Events by Distance

Sprints

Sprints are short running events in athletics and track and field. Races over short distances are among the oldest running competitions. The first 13 editions of the Ancient Olympic Games featured only one event – the stadion race, which was a race from one end of the stadium to the other. There are three sprinting events which are currently held at the Olympics and outdoor World Championships: the 100 metres, 200 metres, and 400 metres. These events have their roots in races of imperial measurements which were later altered to metric: the 100 m evolved from the 100-yard dash, the 200 m distances came from the furlong (or 1/8 of a mile), and the 400 m was the successor to the 440 yard dash or quarter-mile race.

At the professional level, sprinters begin the race by assuming a crouching position in the starting blocks before leaning forward and gradually moving into an upright position as the contest progresses and momentum is gained. Athletes remain in the same lane on the running track throughout all sprinting events, with the sole exception of the 400 m indoors. Races up to 100 m are largely focused upon acceleration to an athlete's maximum speed. All sprints beyond this distance increasingly incorporate an element of endurance. Human physiology dictates that a runner's near-top speed cannot be maintained for more than thirty seconds or so as lactic acid builds up, and leg muscles begin to be deprived of oxygen.

The 60 metres is a common indoor event and it an indoor world championship event. Other less-common events include the 50 metres, 55 metres, 300 metres and 500 metres which are used in some high and collegiate competitions in the United States. The 150 metres, though rarely competed, has a star-studded history: Pietro Mennea set a world best in 1983, Olympic champions Michael Johnson and Donovan Bailey went head-to-head over the distance in 1997, and Usain Bolt improved Mennea's record in 2009.

Middle Distance

Middle distance running events are track races longer than sprints up to 3000 metres. The standard middle distances are the 800 metres, 1500 metres and mile run, although the 3000 metres may also be classified as a middle distance event. The 880 yard run, or half mile, was the forebear to the 800 m distance and it has its roots in competitions in the United Kingdom in the 1830s. The 1500 m came about as a result of running three laps of a 500 m track, which was commonplace in continental Europe in the 1900s.

Long Distance

Examples of longer-distance running events are long distance track races, marathons, ultramarathons, and multiday races.

Animal Locomotion

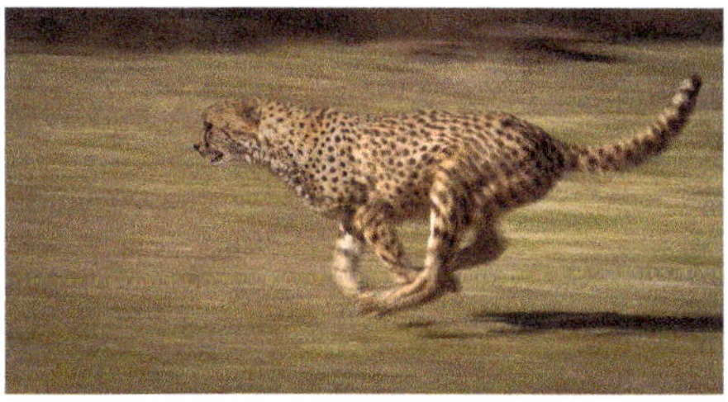

A cheetah chasing prey. In its brief hunting sprints, it is the fastest of all land animals.

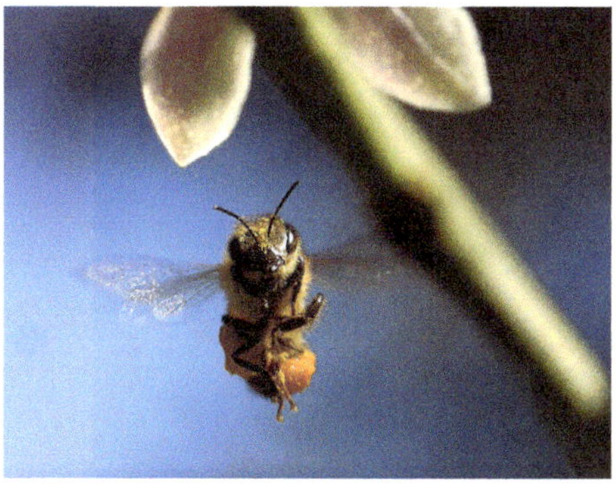

A bee in flight

Animal locomotion, in ethology, is any of a variety of movements or methods that animals use to move from one place to another. Some modes of locomotion are (initially) self-propelled, e.g., running, swimming, jumping, flying, hopping, soaring and gliding. There are also many animal species that depend on their environment for transportation, a type of mobility called passive locomotion, e.g., sailing (some jellyfish), kiting (spiders) and rolling (some beetles and spiders).

Animals move for a variety of reasons, such as to find food, a mate, a suitable microhabitat, or to escape predators. For many animals, the ability to move is essential for survival and, as a result, natural selection has shaped the locomotion methods and mechanisms used by moving organisms. For example, migratory animals that travel vast distances (such as the Arctic tern) typically have a locomotion mechanism that costs very little energy per unit distance, whereas non-migratory animals that must frequently move quickly to escape predators are likely to have energetically costly, but very fast, locomotion.

The anatomical structures that animals use for movement, including cilia, legs, wings, arms, fins, or tails, in various modes and through various media are sometimes referred to as *locomotory organs* or *locomotory structures.*

Etymology

The term "locomotion" is formed in English from Latin *loco* "from a place" (ablative of *locus* "place") + *motio* "motion, a moving".

Locomotion in Different Media

Animals move through, or on, four types of environment: aquatic (in or on water), terrestrial (on ground or other surface, including arboreal, or tree-dwelling), fossorial (underground), and aerial (in the air). Many animals—for example semi-aquatic animals, and diving birds—regularly move through more than one type of medium. In some cases, the surface they move on facilitates their method of locomotion.

Aquatic

Swimming

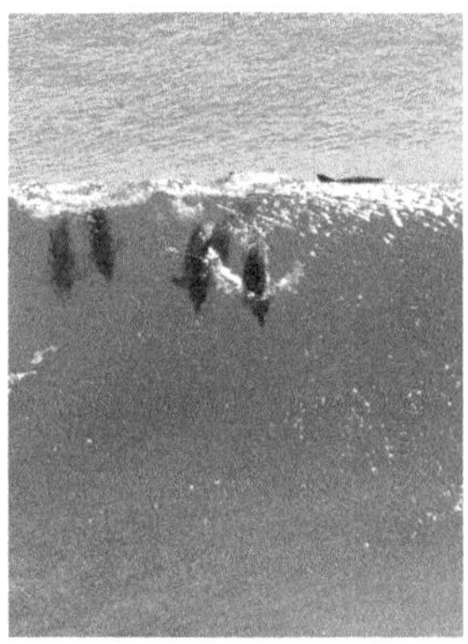

Dolphins surfing

In water, staying afloat is possible using buoyancy. If an animal's body is less dense than water, it can stay afloat. This requires little energy to maintain a vertical position, but requires more energy for locomotion in the horizontal plane compared to less buoyant animals. The drag encountered in water is much greater than in air. Morphology is therefore important for efficient locomotion, which is in most cases essential for basic functions such as catching prey. A fusiform, torpedo-like body form is seen in many aquatic animals, though the mechanisms they use for locomotion are diverse.

The primary means by which fish generate thrust is by oscillating the body from side-to-side, the resulting wave motion ending at a large tail fin. Finer control, such as for slow movements, is often achieved with thrust from pectoral fins (or front limbs in marine mammals). Some fish, e.g. the spotted ratfish (*Hydrolagus colliei*) and batiform fish (electric rays, sawfishes, guitarfishes, skates and stingrays) use their pectoral fins as the primary means of locomotion, sometimes termed labriform swimming. Marine mammals oscillate their body in an up-and-down (dorso-ventral) direction. Other animals, e.g. penguins, diving ducks, move underwater in a manner which has been termed "aquatic flying". Some fish propel themselves without a wave motion of the body, as in the slow-moving seahorses and *Gymnotus*. Other animals, such as cephalopods, use jet propulsion to travel fast, taking in water then squirting it back out in an explosive burst. Other swimming animals may rely predominantly on their limbs, much as humans do when swimming. Though life on land originated from the seas, terrestrial animals have returned to an aquatic lifestyle on several occasions, such as the fully aquatic cetaceans, now very distinct from their terrestrial ancestors.

Dolphins sometimes ride on the bow waves created by boats or surf on naturally breaking waves.

Benthic

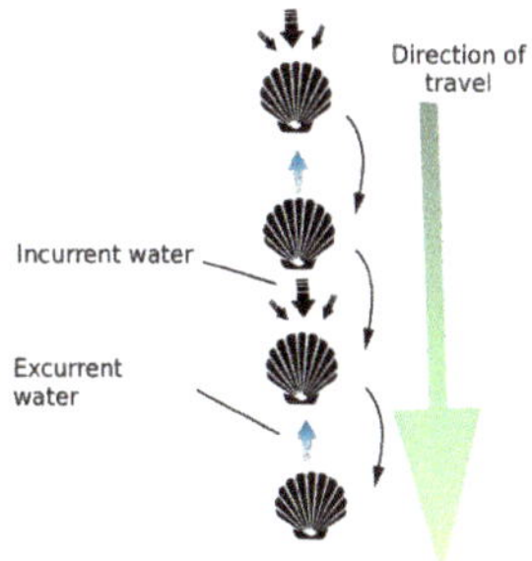

Scallop in jumping motion; these bivalves can also swim.

Benthic locomotion is movement by animals that live on, in, or near the bottom of aquatic environments. In the sea, many animals walk over the seabed. Echinoderms primarily use their tube feet to move about. The tube feet typically have a tip shaped like a suction pad that can create a vacuum through contraction of muscles. This, along with some stickiness from the secretion of mucus, provides adhesion. Waves of tube feet contractions and relaxations move along the adherent surface and the animal moves slowly along. Some sea urchins also use their spines for benthic locomotion.

Crabs typically walk sideways (a behaviour that gives us the word *crabwise*). This is because of the articulation of the legs, which makes a sidelong gait more efficient. However, some crabs walk forwards or backwards, including raninids, *Libinia emarginata* and *Mictyris platycheles*. Some crabs, notably the Portunidae and Matutidae, are also capable of swimming, the Portunidae especially so as their last pair of walking legs are flattened into swimming paddles.

A stomatopod, *Nannosquilla decemspinosa*, can escape by rolling itself into a self-propelled wheel and somersault backwards at a speed of 72 rpm. They can travel more than 2 m using this unusual method of locomotion.

Aquatic Surface

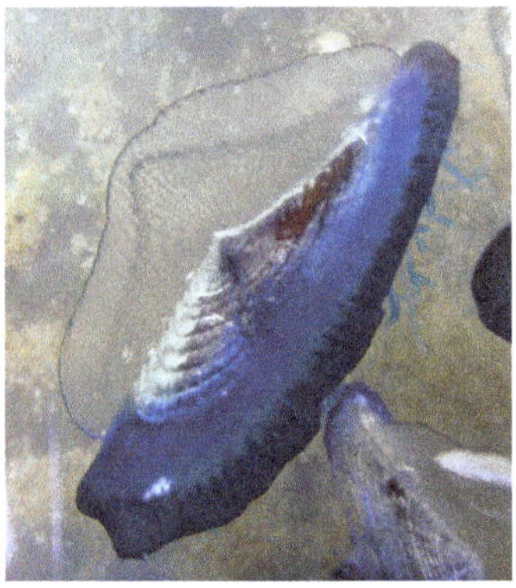

Velella moves by sailing.

Velella, the by-the-wind sailor, is a cnidarian with no means of propulsion other than sailing. A small rigid sail projects into the air and catches the wind. *Velella* sails always align along the direction of the wind where the sail may act as an aerofoil, so that the animals tend to sail downwind at a small angle to the wind.

While larger animals such as ducks can move on water by floating, some small animals move across it without breaking through the surface. This surface locomotion takes advantage of the surface tension of water. Animals that move in such a way include the water strider. Water striders have legs that are hydrophobic, preventing them from interfering with the structure of water. Another form of locomotion (in which the surface layer is broken) is used by the basilisk lizard.

Aerial

Active Flight

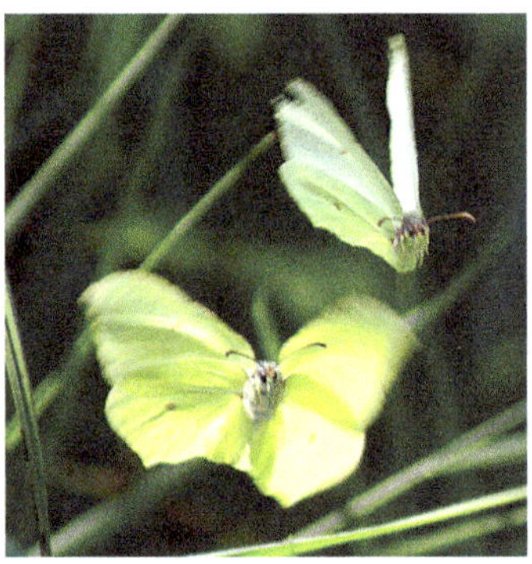

A pair of brimstone butterflies in flight. The female, above, is in fast forward flight with a small angle of attack; the male, below, is twisting his wings sharply upward to gain lift and fly up towards the female.

Gravity is the primary obstacle to flight. Because it is impossible for any organism to have a density as low as that of air, flying animals must generate enough lift to ascend and remain airborne. One way to achieve this is with wings, which when moved through the air generate an upward lift force on the animal's body. Flying animals must be very light to achieve flight, the largest living flying animals being birds of around 20 kilograms. Other structural adaptations of flying animals include reduced and redistributed body weight, fusiform shape and powerful flight muscles; there may also be physiological adaptations. Active flight has independently evolved at least four times, in the insects, pterosaurs, birds, and bats. Insects were the first taxon to evolve flight, approximately 400 million years ago (mya), followed by pterosaurs approximately 220 mya, birds approximately 160 mya, then bats about 60 mya.

Gliding

Rather than active flight, some (semi-) arboreal animals reduce their rate of falling by gliding. Gliding is heavier-than-air flight without the use of thrust; the term "volplaning" also refers to this mode of flight in animals. This mode of flight involves flying a greater distance horizontally than vertically and therefore can be distinguished from a simple descent like a parachute. Gliding has evolved on more occasions than active flight. There are examples of gliding animals in several major taxonomic classes such as the invertebrates (e.g., gliding ants), reptiles (e.g., banded flying snake), amphibians (e.g., flying frog), mammals (e.g., sugar glider, squirrel glider).

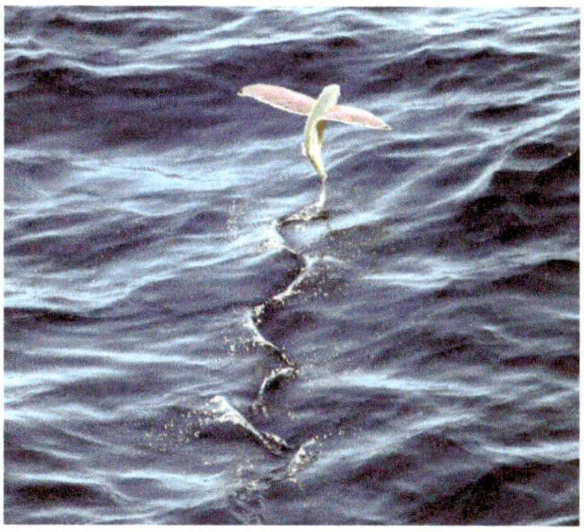

Flying fish taking off

Some aquatic animals also regularly use gliding, for example, flying fish, octopus and squid. The flights of flying fish are typically around 50 meters (160 ft), though they can use updrafts at the leading edge of waves to cover distances of up to 400 m (1,300 ft). To glide upward out of the water, a flying fish moves its tail up to 70 times per second. Several oceanic squid, such as the Pacific flying squid, leap out of the water to escape predators, an adaptation similar to that of flying fish. Smaller squids fly in shoals, and have been observed to cover distances as long as 50 m. Small fins towards the back of the mantle help stabilize the motion of flight. They exit the water by expelling water out of their funnel, indeed some squid have been observed to continue jetting water while airborne providing thrust even after leaving the water. This may make flying squid the only animals with jet-propelled aerial locomotion. The neon flying squid has been observed to glide for distances over 30 m, at speeds of up to 11.2 m/s.

Soaring

Soaring birds can maintain flight without wing flapping, using rising air currents. Many gliding birds are able to "lock" their extended wings by means of a specialized tendon. Soaring birds may alternate glides with periods of soaring in rising air. Five principal types of lift are used: thermals, ridge lift, lee waves, convergences and dynamic soaring.

Examples of soaring flight by birds are the use of:

- Thermals and convergences by raptors such as vultures
- Ridge lift by gulls near cliffs
- Wave lift by migrating birds
- Dynamic effects near the surface of the sea by albatrosses

Ballooning

Ballooning is a method of locomotion used by spiders. Certain silk-producing arthropods, mostly small or young spiders, secrete a special light-weight gossamer silk for ballooning, sometimes traveling great distances at high altitude.

Terrestrial

Forms of locomotion on land include walking, running, hopping or jumping, dragging and crawling or slithering. Here friction and buoyancy are no longer an issue, but a strong skeletal and muscular framework are required in most terrestrial animals for structural support. Each step also requires much energy to overcome inertia, and animals can store elastic potential energy in their tendons to help overcome this. Balance is also required for movement on land. Human infants learn to crawl first before they are able to stand on two feet, which requires good coordination as well as physical development. Humans are bipedal animals, standing on two feet and keeping one on the ground at all times while walking. When running, only one foot is on the ground at any one time at most, and both leave the ground briefly. At higher speeds momentum helps keep the body upright, so more energy can be used in movement.

Jumping

Jumping (saltation) can be distinguished from running, galloping, and other gaits where the entire body is temporarily airborne by the relatively long duration of the aerial phase and high angle of initial launch. Many terrestrial animals use jumping (including hopping or leaping) to escape predators or catch prey—however, relatively few animals use this as a primary mode of locomotion. Those that do include the kangaroo and other macropods, rabbit, hare, jerboa, hopping mouse, and kangaroo rat. Kangaroo rats often leap 2 m and reportedly up to 2.75 m at speeds up to almost 3 m/s (6.7 mph). They can quickly change their direction between jumps. The rapid locomotion of the banner-tailed kangaroo rat may minimize energy cost and predation risk. Its use of a "move-freeze" mode may also make it less conspicuous to nocturnal predators. Frogs are, relative to their size, the best jumpers of all vertebrates. The Australian rocket frog, *Litoria nasuta*, can leap over 2 metres (6 ft 7 in), more than fifty times its body length.

Peristalsis

Other animals move in terrestrial habitats without the aid of legs. Earthworms crawl by a peristalsis, the same rhythmic contractions that propel food through the digestive tract.

Sliding

Due to its low coefficient of friction, ice provides the opportunity for other modes of locomotion. Penguins either waddle on their feet or slide on their bellies across the snow, a movement called *tobogganing*, which conserves energy while moving quickly. Some pinnipeds perform a similar behaviour called *sledding*.

Brachiation

Some animals are specialized for moving on non-horizontal surfaces. One common habitat for such climbing animals is in trees, for example the gibbon is specialized for arboreal movement, traveling rapidly by brachiation. Another case is animals like the snow leopard living on steep rock faces such as are found in mountains. Some light animals are able to climb up smooth sheer surfaces or hang upside down by adhesion. Many insects can do this, though much larger animals such as geckos can also perform similar feats.

Walking and Running

Species have different numbers of legs resulting in large differences in locomotion.

Modern birds, though classified as tetrapods, usually have only two functional legs, which some (e.g., ostrich, emu, kiwi) use as their primary, Bipedal, mode of locomotion. Few modern mammmalian species are habitual bipeds whose normal method of locomotion is two-legged. These include the macropods, kangaroo rats and mice, springhare, hopping mice, pangolins and homininan apes. Bipedalism is rarely found outside terrestrial animals—though at least two types of octopus walk bipedally on the sea floor using two of their arms, so they can use the remaining arms to camouflage themselves as a mat of algae or floating coconut.

There are no three-legged animals—though some macropods, such as kangaroos, that alternate between resting their weight on their muscular tails and their two hind legs, could be looked at as an example of tripedal locomotion in animals.

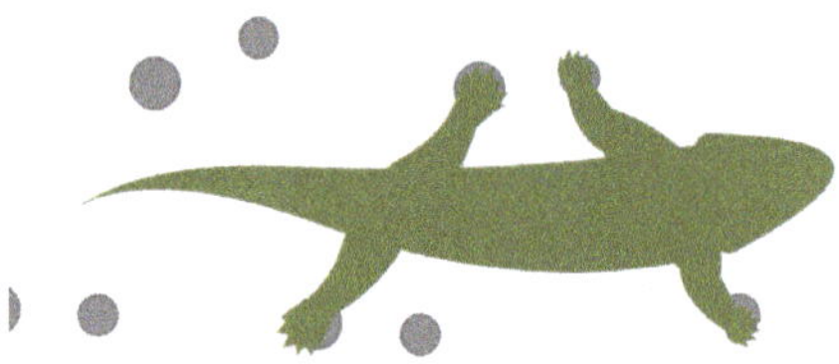
AN EIFELIAN TETRAPOD TRACK AND ITS MAKER
Muz. PGI 1728.II.16 - the Zachełmie quarry, Poland
based on Niedźwiedzki et al. 2010

Devonian tetrapod

Many familiar animals are quadrupedal, walking or running on four legs. A few birds use quadrupedal movement in some circumstances. For example, the shoebill sometimes uses its wings to right itself after lunging at prey. The newly hatched hoatzin bird has claws on its thumb and first finger enabling it to dexterously climb tree branches until its wings are strong enough for sustained flight. These claws are gone by the time the bird reaches adulthood.

A relatively few animals use five limbs for locomotion. Prehensile quadrupeds may use their tail to assist in locomotion and when grazing, the kangaroos and other macropods use their tail to propel themselves forward with the four legs used to maintain balance.

Insects generally walk with six legs—though some insects such as nymphalid butterflies do not use the front legs for walking.

Arachnids have eight legs. Most arachnids lack extensor muscles in the distal joints of their appendages. Spiders and whipscorpions extend their limbs hydraulically using the pressure of their hemolymph. Solifuges and some harvestmen extend their knees by the use of highly elastic thickenings in the joint cuticle. Scorpions, pseudoscorpions and some harvestmen have evolved muscles that extend two leg joints (the femur-patella and patella-tibia joints) at once.

The scorpion *Hadrurus arizonensis* walks by using two groups of legs (left 1, right 2, Left 3, Right 4 and Right 1, Left 2, Right 3, Left 4) in a reciprocating fashion. This alternating tetrapod coordination is used over all walking speeds.

Centipedes and millipedes have many sets of legs that move in metachronal rhythm. Some echinoderms locomote using the many tube feet on the underside of their arms. Although the tube feet resemble suction cups in appearance, the gripping action is a function of adhesive chemicals rather than suction. Other chemicals and relaxation of the ampullae allow for release from the substrate. The tube feet latch on to surfaces and move in a wave, with one arm section attaching to the surface as another releases. Some multi-armed, fast-moving starfish such as the sunflower seastar (*Pycnopodia helianthoides*) pull themselves along with some of their arms while letting others trail behind. Other starfish turn up the tips of their arms while moving, which exposes the sensory tube feet and eyespot to external stimuli. Most starfish cannot move quickly, a typical speed being that of the leather star (*Dermasterias imbricata*), which can manage just 15 cm (6 in) in a minute. Some burrowing species from the genera *Astropecten* and *Luidia* have points rather than suckers on their long tube feet and are capable of much more rapid motion, "gliding" across the ocean floor. The sand star (*Luidia foliolata*) can travel at a speed of 2.8 m (9 ft 2 in) per minute. Sunflower starfish are quick, efficient hunters, moving at a speed of 1 m/min (3.3 ft/min) using 15,000 tube feet.

Many animals temporarily change the number of legs they use for locomotion in different circumstances. For example, many quadrupedal animals switch to bipedalism to reach low-level browse on trees. The genus of *Basiliscus* are arboreal lizards that usually use quadrupedalism in the trees. When frightened, they can drop to water below and run across the surface on their hind limbs at about 1.5 m/s for a distance of approximately 4.5 metres (15 ft) before they sink to all fours and swim. They can also sustain themselves on all fours while "water-walking" to increase the distance travelled above the surface by about 1.3 metres. When cockroaches run rapidly, they rear up on their two hind legs like bipedal humans; this allows them to run at speeds up to 50 body lengths/s, equivalent to a "couple hundred miles per hour, if you scale up to the size of humans". When grazing, kangaroos use a form of pentapedalism (four legs plus the tail) but switch to hopping (bipedalism) when they wish to move at a greater speed.

Powered Cartwheeling

The Moroccan flic-flac spider (*Cebrennus rechenbergi*) uses a series of rapid, acrobatic flic-flac movements of its legs similar to those used by gymnasts, to actively propel itself off the ground, allowing it to move both down and uphill, even at a 40 percent incline. This behaviour is different than other huntsman spiders, such as *Carparachne aureoflava* from the Namib Desert, which uses passive cartwheeling as a form of locomotion. The flic-flac spider can reach speeds of up to 2 m/s using forward or back flips to evade threats.

Subterranean

Some animals move through solids such as soil by burrowing using peristalsis, as in earthworms, or other methods. In loose solids such as sand some animals, such as the golden mole, marsupial mole, and the pink fairy armadillo, are able to move more rapidly, 'swimming' through the loose substrate. Burrowing animals include moles, ground squirrels, naked mole-rats, tilefish, and mole crickets.

Arboreal Locomotion

Arboreal locomotion is the locomotion of animals in trees. Some animals may only scale trees occasionally, while others are exclusively arboreal. These habitats pose numerous mechanical challenges to animals moving through them, leading to a variety of anatomical, behavioural and ecological consequences as well as variations throughout different species. Furthermore, many of these same principles may be applied to climbing without trees, such as on rock piles or mountains. The earliest known tetrapod with specializations that adapted it for climbing trees, was *Suminia*, a synapsid of the late Permian, about 260 million years ago. Some invertebrate animals are exclusively arboreal in habitat, for example, the tree snail.

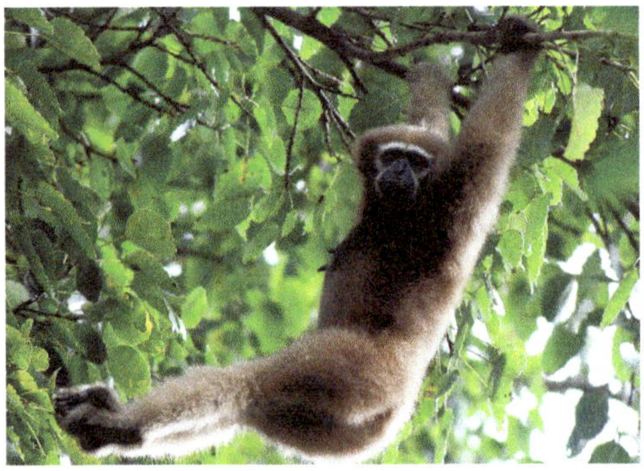

A brachiating gibbon

Brachiation (from *brachium*, Latin for "arm"), is a form of arboreal locomotion in which primates swing from tree limb to tree limb using only their arms. During brachiation, the body is alternately supported under each forelimb. This is the primary means of locomotion for the small gibbons and siamangs of southeast Asia. Some New World monkeys such as spider monkeys and muriquis are "semibrachiators" and move through the trees with a combination of leaping and brachiation. Some New World species also practice suspensory behaviors by using their prehensile tail, which acts as a fifth grasping hand.

Energetics

Animal locomotion requires energy to overcome various forces including friction, drag, inertia and gravity, although the influence of these depends on the circumstances. In terrestrial environments, gravity must be overcome whereas the drag of air has little influence. In aqueous environments, friction (or drag) becomes the major energetic challenge with gravity being less of an influence. Remaining in the aqueous environment, animals with natural buoyancy expend little energy to maintain a vertical position in a water column. Others naturally sink, and must spend energy to remain afloat. Drag is also an energetic influence in flight, and the aerodynamically efficient body shapes of flying birds indicate how they have evolved to cope with this. Limbless organisms moving on land must energetically overcome surface friction, however, they do not usually need to expend significant energy to counteract gravity.

Newton's third law of motion is widely used in the study of animal locomotion: if at rest, to move forwards an animal must push something backwards. Terrestrial animals must push the solid ground, swimming and flying animals must push against a fluid (either water or air). The effect of forces during locomotion on the design of the skeletal system is also important, as is the interaction between locomotion and muscle physiology, in determining how the structures and effectors of locomotion enable or limit animal movement. The energetics of locomotion involves the energy expenditure by animals in moving. Energy consumed in locomotion is not available for other efforts, so animals typically have evolved to use the minimum energy possible during movement. However, in the case of certain behaviors, such as locomotion to escape a predator, performance (such as speed or maneuverability) is more crucial, and such movements may be energetically expensive. Furthermore, animals may use energetically expensive methods of locomotion when environmental conditions (such as being within a burrow) preclude other modes.

The most common metric of energy use during locomotion is the net [also termed "incremental"] cost of transport, defined as the amount of energy (e.g., Joules) needed above baseline metabolic rate to move a given distance. For aerobic locomotion, most animals have a nearly constant cost of transport - moving a given distance requires the same caloric expenditure, regardless of speed. This constancy is usually accomplished by changes in gait. The net cost of transport of swimming is lowest, followed by flight, with terrestrial limbed locomotion being the most expensive per unit distance. However, because of the speeds involved, flight requires the most energy per unit time. This does not mean that an animal that normally moves by running would be a more efficient swimmer; however, these comparisons assume an animal is specialized for that form of motion. Another consideration here is body mass—heavier animals, though using more total energy, require less energy *per unit mass* to move. Physiologists generally measure energy use by the amount of oxygen consumed, or the amount of carbon dioxide produced, in an animal's respiration. In terrestrial animals, the cost of transport is typically measured while they walk or run on a motorized treadmill, either wearing a mask to capture gas exchange or with the entire treadmill enclosed in a metabolic chamber. For small rodents, such as deer mice, the cost of transport has also been measured during voluntary wheel running.

Energetics is important for explaining the evolution of foraging economic decisions in organisms; for example, a study of the African honey bee, *A. m. scutellata*, has shown that honey bees may trade-off the high sucrose content of viscous nectar for the energetic benefits of warmer, less concentrated nectar, which also reduces their consumption and flight time.

Passive Locomotion

Passive locomotion in animals is a type of mobility in which the animal depends on their environment for transportation.

Hydrozoans

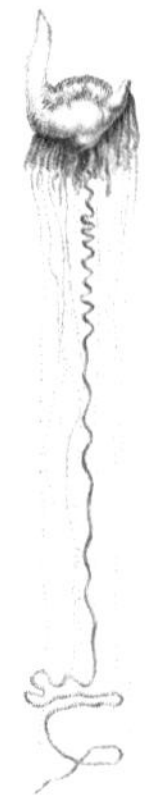

Physalia physalis

The Portuguese man o' war (*Physalia physalis*) lives at the surface of the ocean. The gas-filled bladder, or pneumatophore (sometimes called a "sail"), remains at the surface, while the remainder is submerged. Because the Portuguese man o' war has no means of propulsion, it is moved by a combination of winds, currents, and tides. The sail is equipped with a siphon. In the event of a surface attack, the sail can be deflated, allowing the organism to briefly submerge.

Arachnids

The wheel spider (*Carparachne aureoflava*) is a huntsman spider approximately 20 mm in size and native to the Namib Desert of Southern Africa. The spider escapes parasitic pompilid wasps by flipping onto its side and cartwheeling down sand dunes at speeds of up to 44 turns per second. If the spider is on a sloped dune, its rolling speed may be 1 metre per second.

A spider (usually limited to individuals of a small species), or spiderling after hatching, climbs as high as it can, stands on raised legs with its abdomen pointed upwards ("tiptoeing"), and then releases several silk threads from its spinnerets into the air. These form a triangle-shaped parachute that carries the spider on updrafts of winds, where even the slightest breeze transports it. The Earth's static electric field may also provide lift in windless conditions.

Insects

The larva of *Cicindela dorsalis*, the eastern beach tiger beetle, is notable for its ability to leap into the air, loop its body into a rotating wheel and roll along the sand at a high speed using wind to propel itself. If the wind is strong enough, the larva can cover up to 60 metres (200 ft) in this manner. This remarkable ability may have evolved to help the larva escape predators such as the tiphiid wasp *Methocha*.

Members of the largest subfamily of cuckoo wasps, Chrysidinae, are generally klepto-parasites, laying their eggs in host nests, where their larvae consume the host egg or larva while it is still young. Chrysidines are distinguished from the members of other subfamilies in that most have flattened or concave lower abdomens and can curl into a defensive ball when attacked by a potential host, a process known as conglobation. Protected by hard chitin in this position, they are expelled from the nest without injury and can search for a less hostile host.

Fleas can jump vertically up to 18 cm and horizontally up to 33 cm, however, although this form of locomotion is initiated by the flea, it has little control of the jump - they always jump in the same direction, with very little variation in the trajectory between individual jumps.

Crustaceans

Although stomatopods typically display the standard locomotion types as seen in true shrimp and lobsters, one species, *Nannosquilla decemspinosa*, has been observed flipping itself into a crude wheel. The species lives in shallow, sandy areas. At low tides, *N. decemspinosa* is often stranded by its short rear legs, which are sufficient for locomotion when the body is supported by water, but not on dry land. The mantis shrimp then performs a forward flip in an attempt to roll towards the next tide pool. *N. decemspinosa* has been observed to roll repeatedly for 2 metres (6.6 ft), but they typically travel less than 1 m (3.3 ft). Again, the animal initiates the movement but has little control during its locomotion.

Animal Transport

Some animals change location because they are attached to, or reside on, another animal or moving structure. This is arguably more accurately termed "animal transport".

Remoras

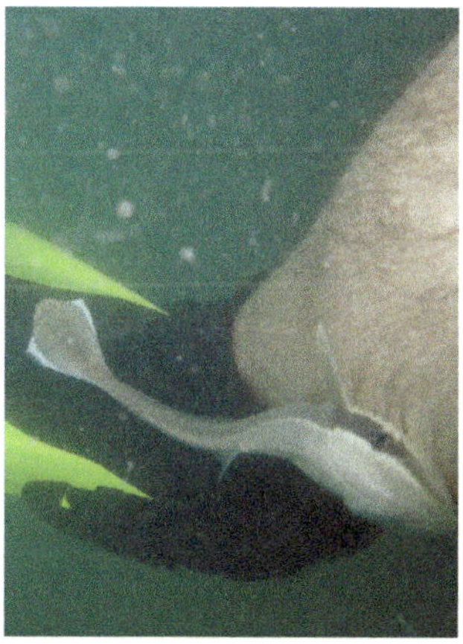

Some remoras, such as this *Echeneis naucrates*, may attach themselves to scuba divers.

Remoras are a family (*Echeneidae*) of ray-finned fish. They grow to 30–90 cm (0.98–2.95 ft) long, and their distinctive first dorsal fins take the form of a modified oval, sucker-like organ with slat-like structures that open and close to create suction and take a firm hold against the skin of larger marine animals. By sliding backward, the remora can increase the suction, or it can release itself by swimming forward. Remoras sometimes attach to small boats. They swim well on their own, with a sinuous, or curved, motion. When the remora reaches about 3 cm (1.2 in), the disc is fully formed and the remora can then attach to other animals. The remora's lower jaw projects beyond the upper, and the animal lacks a swim bladder. Some remoras associate primarily with specific host species. They are commonly found attached to sharks, manta rays, whales, turtles, and dugongs. Smaller remoras also fasten onto fish such as tuna and swordfish, and some small remoras travel in the mouths or gills of large manta rays, ocean sunfish, swordfish, and sailfish. The remora benefits by using the host as transport and protection, and also feeds on materials dropped by the host.

Angler Fish

In some species of anglerfish, when a male finds a female, he bites into her skin, and releases an enzyme that digests the skin of his mouth and her body, fusing the pair down to the blood-vessel level. The male becomes dependent on the female host for survival by receiving nutrients via their shared circulatory system, and provides sperm to the female in return. After fusing, males increase in volume and become much larger relative to free-living males of the species. They live and remain reproductively functional as long as the female lives, and can take part in multiple spawnings. This extreme sexual dimorphism ensures, when the female is ready to spawn, she has a mate immediately available. Multiple males can be incorporated into a single individual female with up to eight males in some species, though some taxa appear to have a one male per female rule.

Parasites

Many endoparasites and ectoparasites, due to their parasitic behaviour, are transported by other animals. For example, tapeworms attach themselves to the inside of the alimentary tracts of other animals and do not locomote within the animal. They do however depend on movement of the host to distribute their eggs.

Other parasites may locomote within, or on, their host, which in turn might be active or stationary. For example, an adult dog flea may crawl about the skin of its sleeping canine host (locomotion), but when the dog awakes and moves, it could be argued the flea is being transported.

Changes between Media

Some animals locomote between different media, e.g., from aquatic to arial. This often requires different modes of locomotion in the different media and may require a distinct transitional locomotor behaviour.

There are a large number of semi-aquatic animals (animals that spend part of their life cycle in water, or generally have part of their anatomy underwater). These represent the major taxons of mammals (e.g., beaver, otter, polar bear), birds (e.g., penguins, ducks), reptiles (e.g., anaconda, bog turtle, marine iguana) and amphibians (e.g., salamanders, frogs, newts).

Fish

Some fish use multiple modes of locomotion. Walking fish may swim freely or at other times "walk" along the ocean or river floor, but not on land (e.g., the flying gurnard – which does not actually fly—and batfishes of the Ogcocephalidae family). Amphibious fish, are fish that are able to leave water for extended periods of time. These fish use a range of terrestrial locomotory modes, such as lateral undulation, tripod-like walking (using paired fins and tail), and jumping. Many of these locomotory modes incorporate multiple combinations of pectoral, pelvic and tail fin movement. Examples include eels, mudskippers and the walking catfish. Flying fish can make powerful, self-propelled leaps out of water into air, where their long, wing-like fins enable gliding flight for considerable distances above the water's surface. This uncommon ability is a natural defense mechanism to evade predators. The flights of flying fish are typically around 50 meters, though they can use updrafts at the leading edge of waves to cover distances of up to 400 m (1,300 ft). They can travel at speeds of more than 70 km/h (43 mph). Maximum altitude is 6 m (20 ft) above the surface of the sea. Some accounts have them landing on ships' decks.

Marine Mammals

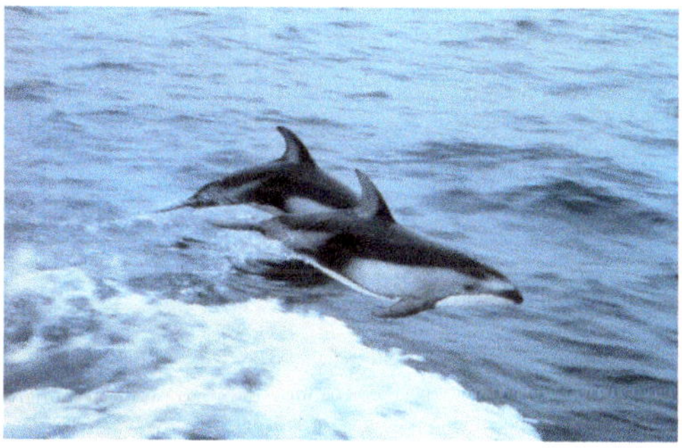

Pacific white-sided dolphins porpoising

When swimming, several marine mammals such as dolphins, porpoises and pinnipeds, frequently leap above the water surface whilst maintaining horizontal locomotion. This is done for various reasons. When travelling, jumping can save dolphins and porpoises energy as there is less friction while in the air. This type of travel is known as "porpoising". Other reasons for dolphins and porpoises performing porpoising include orientation, social displays, fighting, non-verbal communication, entertainment and attempting to dislodge parasites. In pinnipeds, two types of porpoising have been identified. "High porpoising" is most often near (within 100 metres) the shore and is often followed by minor course changes; this may help seals get their bearings on beaching or rafting sites. "Low porpoising" is typically observed relatively far (more than 100 metres) from shore and often aborted in favour of anti-predator movements; this may be a way for seals to maximize sub-surface vigilance and thereby reduce their vulnerability to sharks

Some whales raise their (entire) body vertically out of the water in a behaviour known as "breaching".

Birds

Some semi-aquatic birds use terrestrial locomotion, surface swimming, underwater swimming and flying (e.g., ducks, swans). Diving birds also use diving locomotion (e.g., dippers, aulks). Some birds (e.g., ratites) have lost the primary locomotion of flight. The largest of these, ostriches, when being pursued by a predator, have been known to reach speeds over 70 km/h (43 mph), and can maintain a steady speed of 50 km/h (31 mph), which makes the ostrich the world's fastest two-legged animal: Ostriches can also locomote by swimming. Penguins either waddle on their feet or slide on their bellies across the snow, a movement called *tobogganing*, which conserves energy while moving quickly. They also jump with both feet together if they want to move more quickly or cross steep or rocky terrain. To get onto land, penguins sometimes propel themselves upwards at a great speed to leap out the water.

Changes During the life-cycle

An animal's mode of locomotion may change considerably during its life-cycle. Barnacles are exclusively marine and tend to live in shallow and tidal waters. They have two nektonic (active swimming) larval stages, but as adults, they are sessile (non-motile) suspension feeders. Frequently, adults are found attached to moving objects such as whales and ships, and are thereby transported (passive locomotion) around the oceans.

Function

Animals locomote for a variety of reasons, such as to find food, a mate, a suitable microhabitat, or to escape predators.

Food Procurement

Animals use locomotion in a wide variety of ways to procure food. Terrestrial methods include ambush predation, social predation, grazing. Aquatic methods include filterfeeding, grazing, ram feeding, suction feeding, protrusion and pivot feeding. Other methods include parasitism and parasitoidism.

Methods of Study

A variety of methods and equipment are used to study animal locomotion:

- Treadmills are used to allow animals to walk or run while remaining stationary with respect to external observers. This technique facilitates filming or recordings of physiological information from the animal (e.g., during studies of energetics). Motorized treadmills are also used to measure the endurance capacity (stamina) of animals.
- Racetracks lined with photocells or filmed while animals run along them are used to measure acceleration and maximal sprint speed.
- Kinematics is the study of the motion of an entire animal or parts of its body. It is typically accomplished by placing visual markers at particular anatomical locations on the animal and then recording video of its movement. The video is often captured from multiple angles, with frame rates exceeding 2000 frames per second when capturing high speed movement. The location of each marker is determined for each video frame, and data from multiple views is integrated to give positions of each point through time. Computers are sometimes used to track the markers, although this task must often be performed manually. The kinematic data can be used to determine fundamental motion attributes such as velocity, acceleration, joint angles, and the sequencing and timing of kinematic events. These fundamental attributes can be used to quantify various higher level attributes, such as the physical abilities of the animal (e.g., its maximum running speed, how steep a slope it can climb), neural control of locomotion, gait, and responses to environmental variation. These, in turn, can aid in formulation of hypotheses about the animal or locomotion in general.
- Force plates are platforms, usually part of a trackway, that can be used to measure the magnitude and direction of forces of an animal's step. When used with kinematics and a sufficiently detailed model of anatomy, inverse dynamics solutions can determine the forces not just at the contact with the ground, but at each joint in the limb.
- Electromyography (EMG) is a method of detecting the electrical activity that occurs when muscles are activated, thus determining which muscles an animal uses for a given movement. This can be accomplished either by surface electrodes (usually in large animals) or implanted electrodes (often wires thinner than a human hair). Furthermore, the intensity of electrical activity can correlate to the level of muscle activity, with greater activity implying (though not definitively showing) greater force.
- Sonomicrometry employs a pair of piezoelectric crystals implanted in a muscle or tendon to continuously measure the length of a muscle or tendon. This is

useful because surface kinematics may be inaccurate due to skin movement. Similarly, if an elastic tendon is in series with the muscle, the muscle length may not be accurately reflected by the joint angle.

- Tendon force buckles measure the force produced by a single muscle by measuring the strain of a tendon. After the experiment, the tendon's elastic modulus is determined and used to compute the exact force produced by the muscle. However, this can only be used on muscles with long tendons.
- Particle image velocimetry is used in aquatic and aerial systems to measure the flow of fluid around and past a moving aquatic organism, allowing fluid dynamics calculations to determine pressure gradients, speeds, etc.
- Fluoroscopy allows real-time X-ray video, for precise kinematics of moving bones. Markers opaque to X-rays can allow simultaneous tracking of muscle length.

These methods can be combined. For example, studies frequently combine EMG and kinematics to determine *motor pattern*, the series of electrical and kinematic events that produce a given movement.

Aquatic Locomotion

Aquatic locomotion is biologically propelled motion through a liquid medium. The simplest propulsive systems are composed of cilia and flagella. Swimming has evolved a number of times in a range of organisms including arthropods, fish, molluscs, reptiles, birds, and mammals.

Evolution of Swimming

Swimming evolved a number of times in unrelated lineages. Supposed jellyfish fossils occur in the Ediacaran, but the first free-swimming animals appear in the Early to Middle Cambrian. These are mostly related to the arthropods, and include the Anomalocaridids, which swam by means of lateral lobes in a fashion reminiscent of today's cuttlefish. Cephalopods joined the ranks of the nekton in the late Cambrian, and chordates were probably swimming from the Early Cambrian. Many terrestrial animals retain some capacity to swim, however some have returned to the water and developed the capacities for aquatic locomotion.

Micro-organisms

Ciliates

Ciliates use small flagella called cilia to move through the water. One ciliate will generally have hundreds to thousands of cilia that are densely packed together in arrays.

During movement, an individual cilium deforms using a high-friction power stroke followed by a low-friction recovery stroke. Since there are multiple cilia packed together on an individual organism, they display collective behavior in a metachronal rhythm. This means the deformation of one cilium is in phase with the deformation of its neighbor, causing deformation waves that propagate along the surface of the organism. These propagating waves of cilia are what allow the organism to use the cilia in a coordinated manner to move. A typical example of a ciliated microorganism is the *Paramecium*, a one-celled, ciliated protozoan covered by thousands of cilia. The cilia beating together allow the *Paramecium* to propel through the water at speeds of 500 micrometers per second.

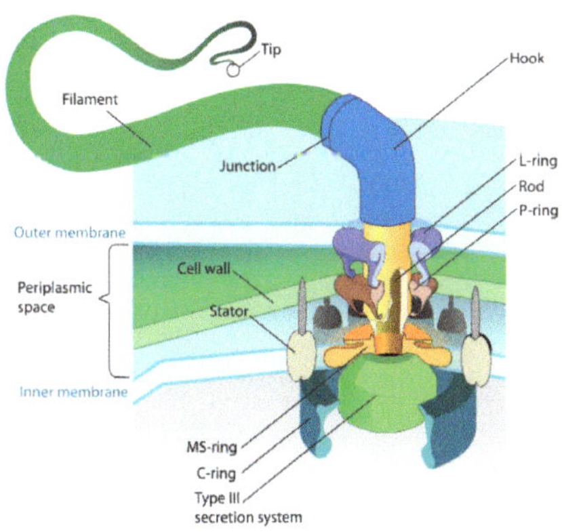

The flagellum of a Gram-negative bacteria is rotated by a molecular motor at its base

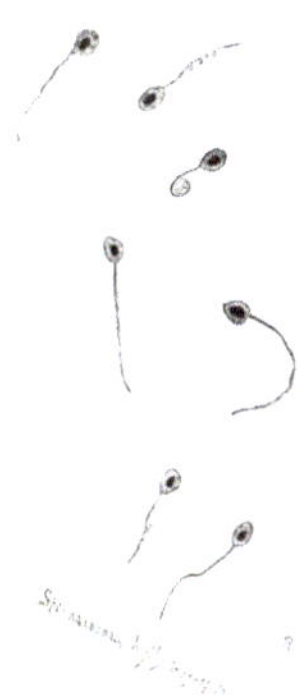

Salmon spermatozoa for artificial propagation

Flagellates

Certain organisms such as bacteria and animal sperm have flagellum which have developed a way to move in liquid environments. A rotary motor model shows that bacteria uses the protons of an electrochemical gradient in order to move their flagella. Torque in the flagella of bacteria is created by particles that conduct protons around the base of the flagellum. The direction of rotation of the flagella in bacteria comes from the occupancy of the proton channels along the perimeter of the flagellar motor.

Movement of sperm is called sperm motility. The middle of the mammalian spermatozoon contains mitochondria that power the movement of the flagellum of the sperm. The motor around the base produces torque, just like in bacteria for movement through the aqueous environment.

Pseudopodia

Movement using a pseudopod is accomplished through increases in pressure at one point on the cell membrane. This pressure increase is the result of actin polymerization between the cortex and the membrane. As the pressure increases the cell membrane is pushed outward creating the pseudopod. When the pseudopod moves outward, the rest of the body is pulled forward by cortical tension. The result is cell movement through the fluid medium. Furthermore, the direction of movement is determined by chemotaxis. When chemoattraction occurs in a particular area of the cell membrane, actin polymerization can begin and move the cell in that direction. An excellent example of an organism that utilizes pseudopods is *Naegleria fowleri.*

Invertebrates

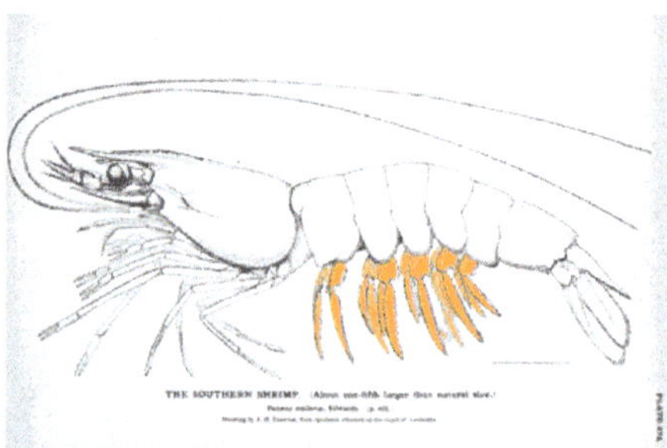

Shrimp paddle with special swimming legs (pleopods)

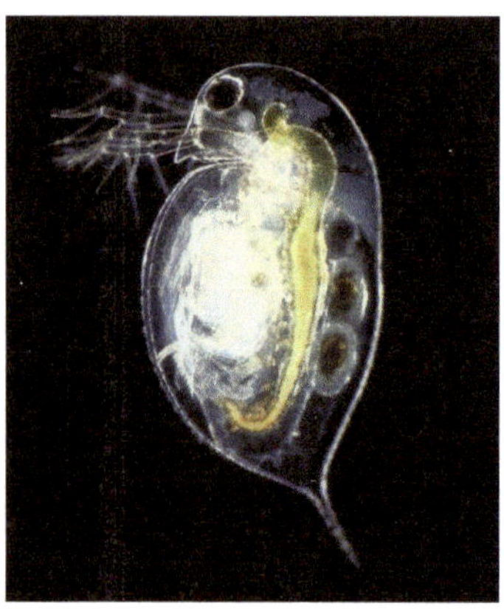

Daphnia swims by beating its antennae

Among the radiata, jellyfish and their kin, the main form of swimming is to flex their cup shaped bodies. All jellyfish are free-swimming, although many of these spend most of their time swimming passively. Passive swimming is akin to gliding; the organism floats, using currents where it can, and does not exert any energy into controlling its position or motion. Active swimming, in contrast, involves the expenditure of energy to travel to a desired location.

In bilateria, there are many methods of swimming. The arrow worms (chaetognatha) undulate their finned bodies, not unlike fish. Nematodes swim by undulating their fin-less bodies. Some Arthropod groups can swim - including many crustaceans. Most crustaceans, such as shrimp, will usually swim by paddling with special swimming legs (pleopods). Swimming crabs swim with modified walking legs (pereiopods). Daphnia, a crustacean, swims by beating its antennae instead.

There are also a number of forms of swimming molluscs. Many free-swimming sea slugs, such as sea angels, flap fin-like structures. Some shelled molluscs, such as scallops can briefly swim by clapping their two shells open and closed. The molluscs most evolved for swimming are the cephalopods.

Among the Deuterostomia, there are a number of swimmers as well. Feather stars can swim by undulating their many arms . Salps move by pumping waters through their gelatinous bodies. The deuterosomes most evolved for swimming are found among the vertebrates, notably the fish.

Jet Propulsion

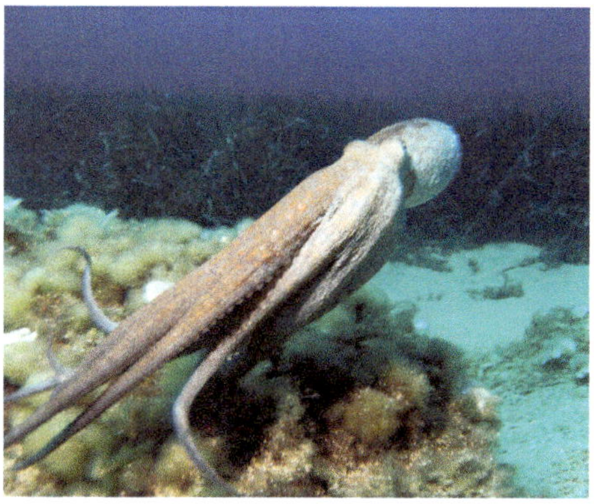

Octopuses swim headfirst, with arms trailing behind

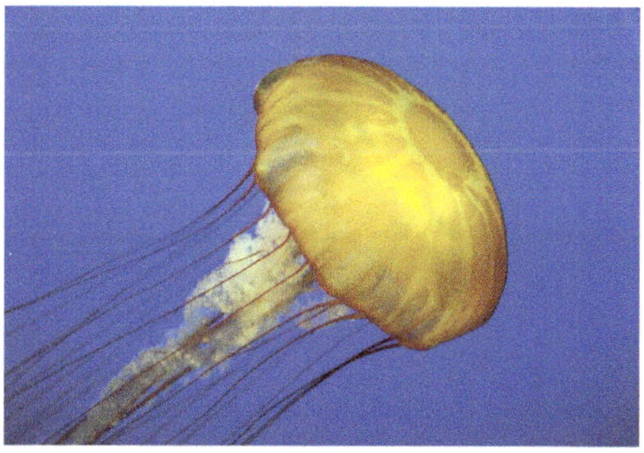

Jellyfish pulsate their bell for a type of jet locomotion

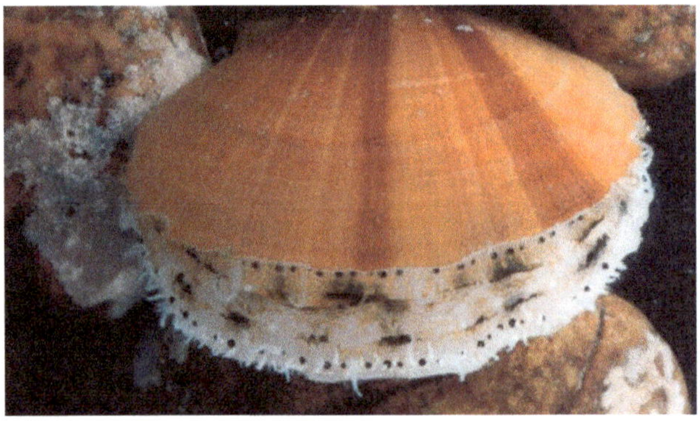

Scallops swim by clapping their two shells open and closed

Jet propulsion is a method of aquatic locomotion where animals fill a muscular cavity and squirt out water to propel them in the opposite direction of the squirting water. Most organisms are equipped with one of two designs for jet propulsion; they can draw water from the rear and expel it from the rear, such as jellyfish, or draw water from front and expel it from the rear, such as salps. Filling up the cavity causes an increase in both the mass and drag of the animal. Because of the expanse of the contracting cavity, the animal's velocity fluctuates as it moves through the water, accelerating while expelling water and decelerating while vacuuming water. Even though these fluctuations in drag and mass can be ignored if the frequency of the jet-propulsion cycles is high enough, jet-propulsion is a relatively inefficient method of aquatic locomotion.

All cephalopods can move by jet propulsion, but this is a very energy-consuming way to travel compared to the tail propulsion used by fish. The relative efficiency of jet propulsion decreases further as animal size increases. Since the Paleozoic, as competition with fish produced an environment where efficient motion was crucial to survival, jet propulsion has taken a back role, with fins and tentacles used to maintain a steady velocity. The stop-start motion provided by the jets, however, continues to be useful for providing bursts of high speed - not least when capturing prey or avoiding predators. Indeed, it makes cephalopods the fastest marine invertebrates, and they can out accelerate most fish. Oxygenated water is taken into the mantle cavity to the gills and through muscular contraction of this cavity, the spent water is expelled through the hyponome, created by a fold in the mantle. Motion of the cephalopods is usually backward as water is forced out anteriorly through the hyponome, but direction can be controlled somewhat by pointing it in different directions. Most cephalopods float (i.e. are neutrally buoyant), so do not need to swim to remain afloat. Squid swim more slowly than fish, but use more power to generate their speed. The loss in efficiency is due to the amount of water the squid can accelerate out of its mantle cavity.

Jellyfish use a one-way water cavity design which generates a phase of continuous cycles of jet-propulsion followed by a rest phase. The Froude efficiency is about 0.09, which indicates a very costly method of locomotion. The metabolic cost of transport for jellyfish is high when compared to a fish of equal mass.

Other jet-propelled animals have similar problems in efficiency. Scallops, which use a similar design to jellyfish, swim by quickly opening and closing their shells, which draws in water and expels it from all sides. This locomotion is used as a means to escape predators such as starfish. Afterwards, the shell acts as a hydrofoil to counteract the scallop's tendency to sink. The Froude efficiency is low for this type of movement, about 0.3, which is why it's used as an emergency escape mechanism from predators. However, the amount of work the scallop has to do is mitigated by the elastic hinge that connects the two shells of the bivalve. Squids swim by drawing water into their mantle cavity and expelling it through their siphon. The Froude efficiency of their jet-propulsion system is around 0.29, which is much lower than a fish of the same mass.

Much of the work done by scallop muscles to close its shell is stored as elastic energy in abductin tissue, which acts as a spring to open the shell. The elasticity causes the work done against the water to be low because of the large openings the water has to enter and the small openings the water has to leave. The inertial work of scallop jet-propulsion is also low. Because of the low inertial work, the energy savings created by the elastic tissue is so small that it's negligible. Medusae can also use their elastic mesoglea to enlarge their bell. Their mantle contains a layer of muscle sandwiched between elastic fibers. The muscle fibers run around the bell circumferentially while the elastic fibers run through the muscle and along the sides of the bell to prevent lengthening. After making a single contraction, the bell vibrates passively at the resonant frequency to refill the bell. However, in contrast with scallops, the inertial work is similar to the hydrodynamic work due to how medusas expel water - through a large opening at low velocity. Because of this, the negative pressure created by the vibrating cavity is lower than the positive pressure of the jet, meaning that inertial work of the mantle is small. Thus, jet-propulsion is shown as an inefficient swimming technique.

Fish

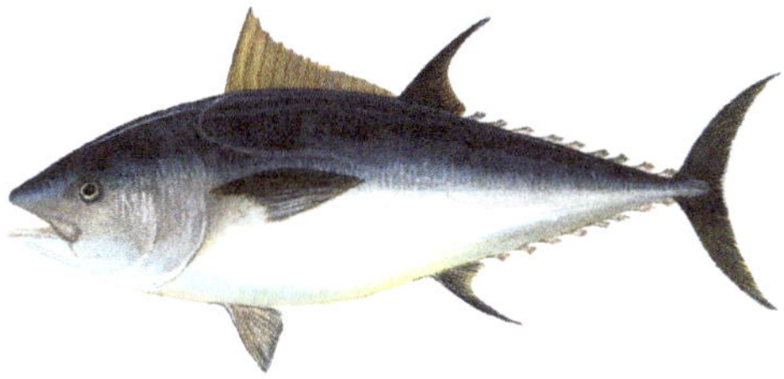

Open water fish, like this Atlantic bluefin tuna, are usually streamlined for straightline speed, with a deeply forked tail and a smooth body shaped like a spindle tapered at both ends.

Many fish swim through water by creating undulations with their bodies or oscillating their fins. The undulations create components of forward thrust complemented by a rearward force, side forces which are wasted portions of energy, and a normal force that is between the forward thrust and side force. Different fish swim by undulating different parts of their bodies. Eel-shaped fish undulate their entire body in rhythmic sequences. Streamlined fish, such as salmon, undulate the caudal portions of their bodies. Some fish, such as sharks, use stiff, strong fins to create dynamic lift and propel themselves. It is common for fish to use more than one form of propulsion, although they will display one dominant mode of swimming Gait changes have even been observed in juvenile reef fish of various sizes. Depending on their needs, fish can rapidly alternate between synchronized fin beats and alternating fin beats

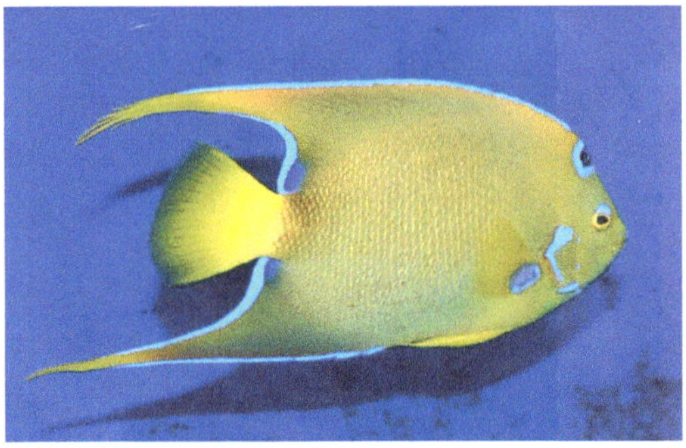

Many reef fish, like this queen angelfish, have a body flattened like a pancake, with pectoral and pelvic fins that act with the flattened body to maximize manoeuvrability.

According to *Guinness World Records 2009*, *H. zosterae* (the dwarf seahorse) is the slowest moving fish, with a top speed of about 5 feet (150 cm) per hour. They swim very poorly, rapidly fluttering a dorsal fin and using pectoral fins (located behind their eyes) to steer. Seahorses have no caudal fin.

Body-caudal Fin (BCF) Propulsion

- Anguilliform: Anguilliform swimmers are typically slow swimmers. They undulate the majority of their body and use their head as the fulcrum for the load they are moving. At any point during their undulation, their body has an amplitude between 0.5-1.0 wavelengths. The amplitude that they move their body through allows them to swim backwards. Anguilliform locomotion is usually seen in fish with long, slender bodies like eels, lampreys, oarfish, and a number of catfish species.

- Subcarangiform, Carangiform, Thunniform: These swimmers undulate the posterior half of their body and are much faster than anguilliform swimmers. At any point while they are swimming, a wavelength <1 can be seen in the undulation pattern of the body. Some Carangiform swimmers include nurse sharks, bamboo sharks, and reef sharks. Thunniform swimmers are very fast and some common Thunniform swimmers include tuna, white sharks, salmon, jacks, and mako sharks. Thunniform swimmers only undulate their high aspect ratio caudal fin, so they are usually very stiff to push more water out of the way.

- Ostraciiform: Ostraciiform swimmers oscillate their caudal region, making them relatively slow swimmers. Boxfish, torpedo rays, and momyrs employ Ostraciiform locomotion. The cow fish uses Osctraciiform locomotion to hover in the water column.

Median Paired Fin (MPF) Propulsion

- Tetraodoniform, Balistiform, Diodontiform: These swimmers oscillate their median fins. They are typically slow swimmers, and some notable examples include the oceanic sunfish (which has extremely modified anal and dorsal fins), puffer fish, and triggerfish.
- Rajiform, Amiiform, Gymnotiform: This locomotory mode is accomplished by undulation of the pectoral and median fins. During their undulation pattern, a wavelength >1 can be seen in their fins. They are typically slow to moderate swimmers, and some examples include rays, bowfin, and knife fishes. The black ghost knife fish is a Gymnotiform swimmer that has a very long ventral ribbon fin. Thrust is produced by passing waves down the ribbon fin while the body remains rigid. This also allows the ghost knife fish to swim in reverse.
- Labriform: Labriform swimmers are also slow swimmers. They oscillate their pectoral fins to create thrust. Oscillating fins create thrust when a starting vortex is shed from the trailing edge of the fin. As the foil departs from the starting vortex, the effect of that vortex diminishes, while the bound circulation remains, producing lift. Labriform swimming can be viewed as continuously starting and stopping. Wrasses and surf perch are common Labriform swimmers

Hydrofoils

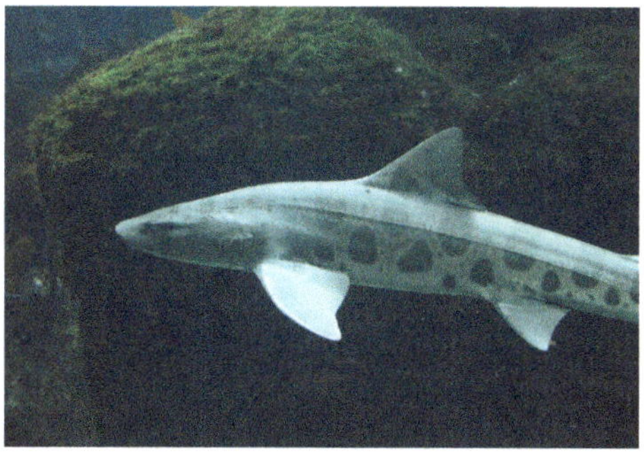

The leopard shark angles its pectoral fins so they behave as hydrofoils to control the animal's pitch.

Hydrofoils, or fins, are used to push against the water to create a normal force to provide thrust, propelling the animal through water. Sea turtles and penguins beat their paired hydrofoils to create lift. Some paired fins, such as pectoral fins on leopard sharks, can be angled at varying degrees to allow the animal to rise, fall, or maintain its level in the water column. The reduction of fin surface area helps to minimize drag, and therefore increase efficiency. Regardless of size of the animal, at any particular speed, maximum possible lift is proportional to (wing area) x $(\text{speed})^2$. Dolphins and whales have large, horizontal caudal hydrofoils, while many fish and sharks have vertical caudal hydrofoils. Porpoising (seen in cetaceans, penguins, and pinnipeds) may save energy if they are moving fast. Since drag increases with speed, the work required to swim unit distance is greater at higher speeds, but the work needed to jump unit distance is independent of speed. Seals propel themselves through the water with their caudal tail, while sea lions create thrust solely with their pectoral flippers.

Drag Powered Swimming

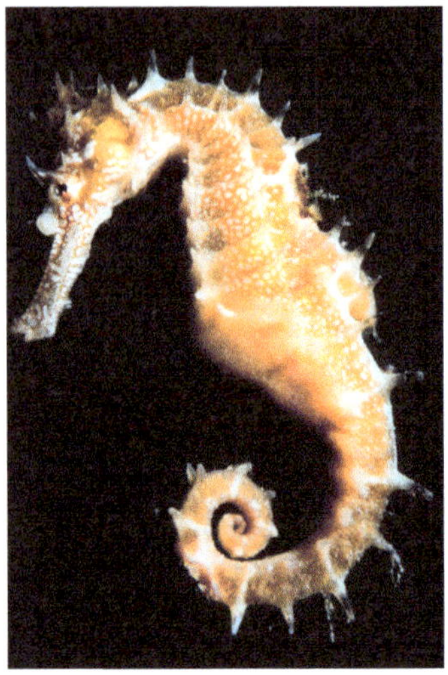

The slowest-moving fishes are the sea horses, often found in reefs.

As with moving through any fluid, friction is created when molecules of the fluid collide with organism. The collision causes drag against moving fish, which is why many fish are streamlined in shape. Streamlined shapes work to reduce drag by orienting elongated objects parallel to the force of drag, therefore allowing the current to pass over and taper off the end of the fish. This streamlined shape allows for more efficient use of energy locomotion. Some flat-shaped fish can take advantage of pressure drag by having a flat bottom surface and curved top surface. The pressure drag created allows for the upward lift of the fish.

Appendages of aquatic organisms propel them in two main and biomechanically extreme mechanisms. Some use lift powered swimming, which can be compared to flying as appendages flap like wings, and reduce drag on the surface of the appendage. Others use drag powered swimming, which can be compared to oars rowing a boat, with movement in a horizontal plane, or paddling, with movement in the parasagittal plane.

Drag swimmers use a cyclic motion where they push water back in a power stroke, and return their limb forward in the return or recovery stroke. When they push water directly backwards, this moves their body forward, but as they return their limbs to the starting position, they push water forward, which will thus pull them back to some degree, and so opposes the direction that the body is heading. This opposing force is called drag. The return-stroke drag causes drag swimmers to employ different strategies than lift swimmers. Reducing drag on the return stroke is essential for optimizing efficiency. For example, ducks paddle through the water spreading the webs of their feet as they move water back, and then when they return their feet to the front they pull their webs together to reduce the subsequent pull of water forward. The legs of water beetles have little hairs which spread out to catch up and move water back in the power stroke, but lay flat as the appendage moves forward in the return stroke. Also, the water beetle's legs have a side that is wider and is held perpendicular to the motion when pushing backward, but the leg is then rotated when the limb is to return forward, so that the thinner side will catch up less water.

Drag swimmers experience a lessened efficiency in swimming due to resistance which affects their optimum speed. The less drag a fish experiences, the more it will be able to maintain higher speeds. Morphology of the fish can be designed to reduce drag, such as streamlining the body. The cost of transport is much higher for the drag swimmer, and when deviating from its optimum speed, the drag swimmer is energetically strained much more than the lift swimmer. There are natural processes in place to optimize energy use, and it is thought that adjustments of metabolic rates can compensate in part for mechanical disadvantages.

Semi-aquatic animals compared to fully aquatic animals exhibit exacerbation of drag. Design that allows them to function out of the water limits the efficiency possible to be reached when in the water. In water swimming at the surface exposes them to resistive wave drag and is associated with a higher cost than submerged swimming. Swimming below the surface exposes them to resistance due to return strokes and pressure, but primarily friction. Frictional drag is due to fluid viscosity and morphology characteristics. Pressure drag is due to the difference of water flow around the body and is also affected by body morphology. Semi-aquatic organisms encounter increased resistive forces when in or out of the water, as they are not specialized for either habitat. The morphology of otters and beavers, for example, must meet needs for both environments. Their fur decreases streamlining and creates additional drag. The platypus may be a good example of an intermediate between drag and lift swimmers because it has been shown to have a rowing mechanism which is similar to lift-based pectoral oscillation. The limbs of semi-aquatic organisms are reserved for use on land and using them in water not only increases the cost of locomotion, but limits them to drag-based modes. Although they are less efficient, drag swimmers are able to produce more thrust at low speeds than lift swimmers. They are also thought to be better for maneuverability due to the large thrust produced.

Amphibians

Most of the Amphibia have a larval state, which has inherited anguilliform motion, and a laterally compressed tail to go with it, from fish ancestors. The corresponding tetrapod adult forms, even in the tail-retaining sub-class Urodeles, are sometimes aquatic to only a negligible extent (as in the genus Salamandra, whose tail has lost its suitability for aquatic propulsion), but the majority of Urodeles, from the newts to the giant salamander Megalobatrachus, retain a laterally compressed tail for a life that is aquatic to a considerable degree, which can use in a carangiform motion.

Of the tailless amphibians (the frogs and toads of the sub-class Anura) the majority are aquatic to an insignificant extent in adult life, but in that considerable minority that are mainly aquatic we encounter for the first time the problem of adapting the tailless-tetrapod structure for aquatic propulsion. The mode that they use is unrelated to any used by fish. With their flexible back legs and webbed feet they execute something close to the leg movements of a human 'breast stroke,' rather more efficiently because the legs are better streamlined.

Reptiles

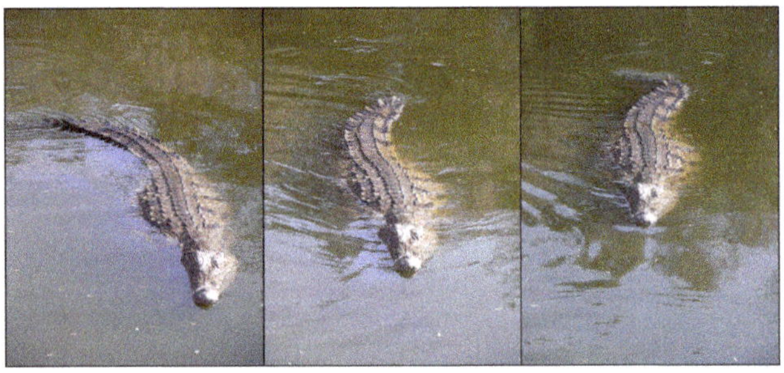

Nile crocodile (*Crocodylus niloticus*) swimming

From the point of view of aquatic propulsion, the descent of modern members of the class Reptilia from archaic tailed Amphibia is most obvious in the case of the order Crocodilia (crocodiles and alligators), which use their deep, laterally compressed tails in an essentially carangiform mode of propulsion.

Terrestrial snakes, in spite of their 'bad' hydromechanical shape with roughly circular cross-section and gradual posterior taper, swim fairly readily when required, by an anguilliform propulsion

Cheloniidae (true turtles) have found a beautiful solution to the problem of tetrapod swimming through the development of their forelimbs into flippers of high-aspect-ratio wing shape, with which they imitate a bird's propulsive mode more accurately than do the eagle-rays themselves.

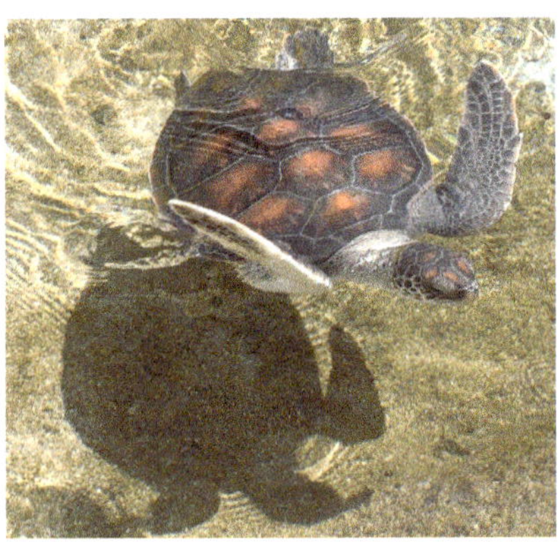

Immature Hawaiian green sea turtle in shallow waters

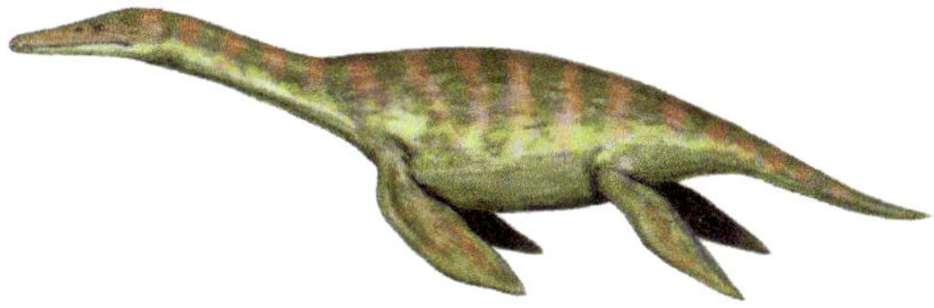

Macroplata

Fin and Flipper Locomotion

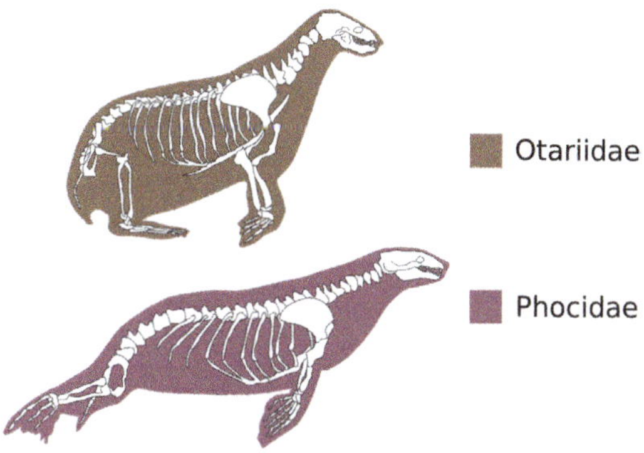

Comparative skeletal anatomy of a typical otariid seal and a typical phocid seal

Aquatic reptiles such as sea turtles and extinct species like Pliosauroids predominantly use their pectoral flippers to propel themselves through the water and their pelvic flippers for maneuvering. During swimming they move their pectoral flippers in a dorso-ventral motion, causing forward motion. During swimming, they rotate their front flippers to decrease drag through the water column and increase efficiency. Newly hatched sea turtles exhibit several behavioral skills that help orientate themselves towards the ocean as well as identifying the transition from sand to water. If rotated in the pitch, yaw or roll direction, the hatchlings are capable of counteracting the forces acting upon them by correcting with either their pectoral or pelvic flippers and redirecting themselves towards the open ocean.

Among mammals otariids (fur seals) swim primarily with their front flippers, using the rear flippers for steering, and phocids (true seals) move the rear flippers laterally, pushing the animal through the water.

Escape Reactions

Some arthropods, such as lobsters and shrimps, can propel themselves backwards quickly by flicking their tail, known as lobstering or the caridoid escape reaction.

Varieties of fish, such as teleosts, also use fast-starts to escape from predators. Fast-starts are characterized by the muscle contraction on one side of the fish twisting the fish into a C-shape. Afterwards, muscle contraction occurs on the opposite side to allow the fish to enter into a steady swimming state with waves of undulation traveling alongside the body. The power of the bending motion comes from fast-twitch muscle fibers located in the central region of the fish. The signal to perform this contraction comes from a set of Mauthner cells which simultaneously send a signal to the muscles on one side of the fish. Mauthner cells are activated when something startles the fish and can be activated by visual or sound-based stimuli.

Fast-starts are split up into three stages. Stage one, which is called the preparatory stroke, is characterized by the initial bending to a C-shape with small delay caused by hydrodynamic resistance. Stage two, the propulsive stroke, involves the body bending rapidly to the other side, which may occur multiple times. Stage three, the rest phase, cause the fish to return to normal steady-state swimming and the body undulations begin to cease. Large muscles located closer to the central portion of the fish are stronger and generate more force than the muscles in the tail. This asymmetry in muscle composition causes body undulations that occur in Stage 3. Once the fast-start is completed, the position of the fish has been shown to have a certain level of unpredictability, which helps fish survive against predators.

The rate at which the body can bend is limited by resistance contained in the inertia of each body part. However, this inertia assists the fish in creating propulsion as a result of the momentum created against the water. The forward propulsion created from C-starts, and steady-state swimming in general, is a result of the body of the fish pushing against the water. Waves of undulation create rearward momentum against the water providing the forward thrust required to push the fish forward.

Efficiency

The Froude propulsion efficiency is defined as the ratio of power output to the power input:

$$nf = 2U_1 / (U_1 + U_2)$$

where U1 = free stream velocity and U2 = jet velocity. A good efficiency for carangiform propulsion is between 50 and 80%.

Minimizing Drag

Pressure differences occur outside the boundary layer of swimming organisms due to disrupted flow around the body. The difference on the up- and down-stream surfaces of the body is pressure drag, which creates a downstream force on the object. Frictional drag, on the other hand, is a result of fluid viscosity in the boundary layer. Higher turbulence causes greater frictional drag.

Reynolds number (Re) is the measure of the relationships between inertial and viscous forces in flow ((animal's length x animal's velocity)/kinematic viscosity of the fluid).

Turbulent flow can be found at higher Re values, where the boundary layer separates and creates a wake, and laminar flow can be found at lower Re values, when the boundary layer separation is delayed, reducing wake and kinetic energy loss to opposing water momentum.

The body shape of a swimming organism affects the resulting drag. Long, slender bodies reduce pressure drag by streamlining, while short, round bodies reduce frictional drag; therefore, the optimal shape of an organism depends on its niche. Swimming organisms with a fusiform shape are likely to experience the greatest reduction in both pressure and frictional drag.

Wing shape also affects the amount of drag experienced by an organism, as with different methods of stroke, recovery of the pre-stroke position results in the accumulation of drag.

High-speed ram ventilation creates laminar flow of water from the gills along the body of an organism.

The secretion of mucus along the organism's body surface, or the addition of long-chained polymers to the velocity gradient, can reduce frictional drag experienced by the organism.

Buoyancy

Many aquatic/marine organisms have developed organs to compensate for their weight and control their buoyancy in the water. These structures, make the density of their bodies very close to that of the surrounding water. Some hydrozoans, such as siphonophores, has gas-filled floats; the Nautilus, Sepia, and Spirula (Cephalopods) have chambers of gas within their shells; and most teleost fish and many lantern fish (Myctophidae) are equipped with swim bladders. Many aquatic and marine organisms may also be composed of low-density materials. Deep-water teleosts, which do not have a swim bladder, have few lipids and proteins, deeply ossified bones, and watery tissues that maintain their buoyancy. Some sharks' livers are composed of low-density lipids, such as hydrocarbon squalene or wax esters (also found in Myctophidae without swim bladders), which provide buoyancy.

Swimming animals that are denser than water must generate lift or adapt a benthic lifestyle. Movement of the fish to generate hydrodynamic lift is necessary to prevent sinking. Often, their bodies act as hydrofoils, a task that is more effective in flat-bodied fish. At a small tilt angle, the lift is greater for flat fish than it is for fish with narrow bodies. Narrow-bodied fish use their fins as hydrofoils while their bodies remain horizontal. In sharks, the heterocercal tail shape drives water downward, creating a counteracting upward force while thrusting the shark forward. The lift generated is assisted by the pectoral fins and upward-angle body positioning. It is supposed that tunas primarily use their pectoral fins for lift.

Buoyancy maintenance is metabolically expensive. Growing and sustaining a buoyancy organ, adjusting the composition of biological makeup, and exerting physical strain to stay in motion demands large amounts of energy. It is proposed that lift may be physically generated at a lower energy cost by swimming upward and gliding downward, in a "climb and glide" motion, rather than constant swimming on a plane.

Temperature

Temperature can also greatly affect the ability of aquatic organisms to move through water. This is because temperature not only affects the properties of the water, but also the organisms in the water, as most have an ideal range specific to their body and metabolic needs.

Q10 (temperature coefficient), the factor by which a rate increases at a 10 °C increase in temperature, is used to measure how organisms' performance relies on temperature. Most have increased rates as water becomes warmer, but some have limits to this and others find ways to alter such effects, such as by endothermy or earlier recruitment of faster muscle.

For example, *Crocodylus porosus*, or estuarine crocodiles, were found to increase swimming speed from 15 °C to 23 °C and then to have peak swimming speed from 23 °C to 33 °C. However, performance began to decline as temperature rose beyond that point, showing a limit to the range of temperatures at which this species could ideally perform.

Submergence

The more of the animal's body that is submerged while swimming, the less energy it uses. Swimming on the surface requires two to three times more energy than when completely submerged. This is because of the bow wave that is formed at the front when the animal is pushing the surface of the water when swimming, creating extra drag.

Secondary Evolution

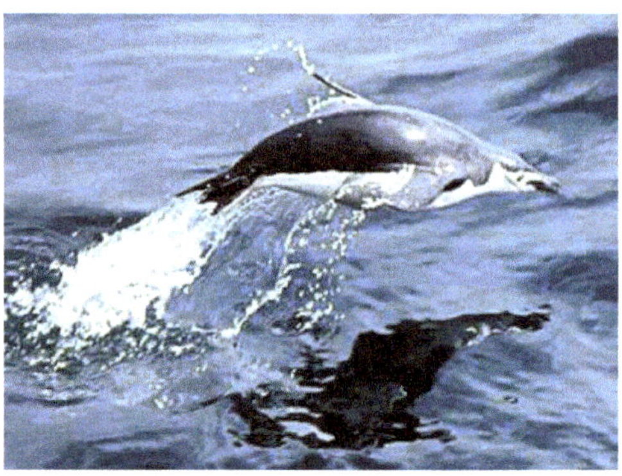

Chinstrap penguin leaping over water

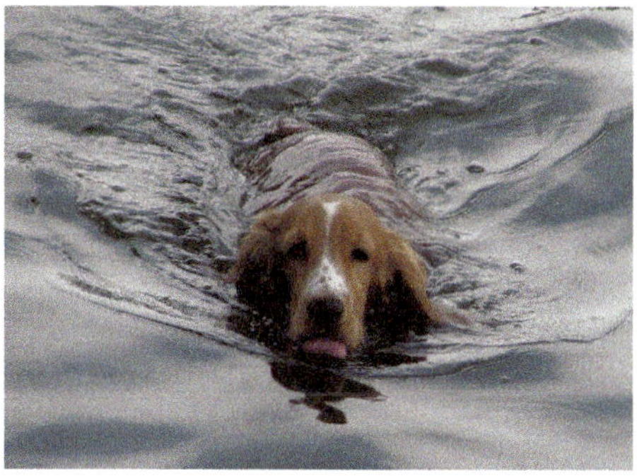

Swimming dog

While tetrapods lost many of their natural adaptations to swimming when they evolved onto the land, many have re-evolved the ability to swim or have indeed returned to a completely aquatic lifestyle.

Primarily or exclusively aquatic animals have re-evolved from terrestrial tetrapods multiple times: examples include amphibians such as newts, reptiles such as crocodiles, sea turtles, ichthyosaurs, plesiosaurs and mosasaurs, marine mammals such as whales, seals and otters, and birds such as penguins. Many species of snakes are also aquatic and live their entire lives in the water. Among invertebrates, a number of insect species have adaptations for aquatic life and locomotion. Examples of aquatic insects include dragonfly larvae, water boatmen, and diving beetles. There are also aquatic spiders, although they tend to prefer other modes of locomotion under water than swimming proper.

Even though primarily terrestrial tetrapods have lost many of their adaptations to swimming, the ability to swim has been preserved or re-developed in many of them. It may never have been completely lost.

Examples are: Some breeds of dog swim recreationally. Umbra, a world record-holding dog, can swim 4 miles (6.4 km) in 73 minutes, placing her in the top 25% in human long-distance swimming competitions. Although most cats hate water, adult cats are good swimmers. The fishing cat is one wild species of cat that has evolved special adaptations for an aquatic or semi-aquatic lifestyle – webbed digits. Tigers and some individual jaguars are the only big cats known to go into water readily, though other big cats, including lions, have been observed swimming. A few domestic cat breeds also like swimming, such as the Turkish Van.

Horses, moose, and elk are very powerful swimmers, and can travel long distances in the water. Elephants are also capable of swimming, even in deep waters. Eyewitnesses have confirmed that camels, including dromedary and Bactrian camels, can swim, despite the fact that there is little deep water in their natural habitats.

Both domestic and wild rabbits can swim. Domestic rabbits are sometimes trained to swim as a circus attraction. A wild rabbit famously swam in an apparent attack on U.S. President Jimmy Carter's boat when it was threatened in its natural habitat.

The guinea pig (or cavy) is noted as having an excellent swimming ability. Mice can swim quite well. They do panic when placed in water, but many lab mice are used in the Morris water maze, a test to measure learning. When mice swim, they use their tails like flagella and kick with their legs.

Many snakes are excellent swimmers as well. Large adult anacondas spend the majority of their time in the water, and have difficulty moving on land.

Many monkeys can naturally swim and some, like the proboscis monkey, crab-eating macaque, and rhesus macaque swim regularly.

Human Swimming

Swimming has been known amongst humans since prehistoric times; the earliest record of swimming dates back to Stone Age paintings from around 7,000 years ago. Competitive swimming started in Europe around 1800 and was part of the first modern 1896 Summer Olympics in Athens, though not in a form comparable to the contemporary events. It was not until 1908 that regulations were implemented by the International Swimming Federation to produce competitive swimming.

Flying and Gliding Animals

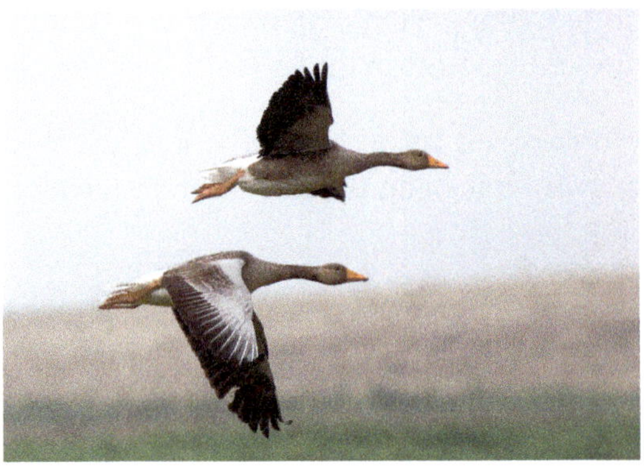

Greylag geese (*Anser anser*). Birds are one of only four taxonomic groups to have evolved powered flight.

A number of animals have evolved aerial locomotion, either by powered flight or by gliding. Flying and gliding animals (*volant* animals) have evolved separately many times, without any single ancestor. Flight has evolved at least four times, in the insects, pterosaurs, birds, and bats. Gliding has evolved on many more occasions. Usually the development is to aid canopy animals in getting from tree to tree, although there are other possibilities. Gliding, in particular, has evolved among rainforest animals, especially in the rainforests in Asia (most especially Borneo) where the trees are tall and widely spaced. Several species of aquatic animals, and a few amphibians have also evolved to acquire this gliding flight ability, typically as a means of evading predators.

Types

Animal aerial locomotion can be divided into two categories—powered and unpowered. In unpowered modes of locomotion, the animal uses on aerodynamics forces exerted on the body due to wind or falling through the air. In powered flight, the animal uses muscular power to generate aerodynamic forces. Animals using unpowered aerial locomotion cannot maintain altitude and speed due to unopposed drag, while animals using powered flight can maintain steady, level flight as long as their muscles are capable of doing so.

Unpowered

These modes of locomotion typically require an animal start from a raised location, converting that potential energy into kinetic energy and using aerodynamic forces to control trajectory and angle of descent. Energy is continually lost to drag without being replaced, thus these methods of locomotion have limited range and duration.

- Falling: decreasing altitude under the force of gravity, using no adaptations to increase drag or provide lift.
- Parachuting: falling at an angle greater than 45° from the horizontal with adaptations to increase drag forces. Very small animals may be carried up by the wind. Some gliding animals may use their gliding membranes for drag rather than lift, to safely descend.
- Gliding flight: falling at an angle less than 45° from the horizontal with lift from adapted aerofoil membranes. This allows slowly falling directed horizontal movement, with streamlining to decrease drag forces for aerofoil efficiency and often with some maneuverability in air. Gliding animals have a lower aspect ratio (wing length/breadth) than true flyers.

Powered Flight

Powered flight has evolved only four times (in birds, bats, pterosaurs, and insects). It uses muscular power to generate aerodynamic forces and to replace energy lost to drag.

- Flapping: moving wings to produce lift and thrust. May ascend without the aid of the wind, as opposed to gliders and parachuters.

Externally Powered

Ballooning and soaring are not powered by muscle, but rather by external aerodynamic sources of energy: the wind and rising thermals, respectively. Both can continue as long as the source of external power is present. Soaring is typically only seen in species capable of powered flight, as it requires extremely large wings.

- Ballooning: being carried up into the air from the aerodynamic effect on long strands of silk in the wind. Certain silk-producing arthropods, mostly small or young spiders, secrete a special light-weight gossamer silk for ballooning, sometimes traveling great distances at high altitude.
- Soaring: gliding in rising or otherwise moving air that requires specific physiological and morphological adaptations that can sustain the animal aloft without flapping its wings. The rising air is due to thermals, ridge lift or other meteorological features. Under the right conditions, soaring creates a gain of altitude without expending energy. Large wingspans are needed for efficient soaring.

Many species will use multiple of these modes at various times; a hawk will use powered flight to rise, then soar on thermals, then descend via free-fall to catch its prey.

Evolution and Ecology

Gliding and Parachuting

While gliding occurs independently from powered flight, it has some ecological advantages of its own. Gliding is a very energy-efficient way of travelling from tree to tree. An argument made is that many gliding animals eat low energy foods such as leaves and are restricted to gliding because of this, whereas flying animals eat more high energy foods such as fruits, nectar, and insects. In contrast to flight, gliding has evolved independently many times (more than a dozen times among extant vertebrates), however these groups have not radiated nearly as much as have groups of flying animals.

Worldwide, the distribution of gliding animals is uneven as most inhabit rain forests in Southeast Asia. (Despite seemingly suitable rain forest habitats, few gliders are found in India or New Guinea and none in Madagascar.) Additionally, a variety of gliding vertebrates are found in Africa, a family of hylids (flying frogs) lives in South America and several species of gliding squirrels are found in the forests of northern Asia and North America. Various factors produce these disparities. In the forests of Southeast Asia, the dominant canopy trees (usually dipterocarps) are taller than the canopy trees of the other forests. A higher start provides a competitive advantage of further glides and farther travel. Gliding predators may more efficiently search for prey. The lower abundance of insect and small vertebrate prey for carnivorous animals (such as lizards) in Asian forests (In Australia, many mammals (and all mammalian gliders) possess, to some extent, prehensile tails.

An abundance of lianas (woody vines) may obstruct gliders but aid climbers with prehensile tails. The differing populations may relate to the prevalence in South America (compared to Africa or Southeast Asia) of animals with prehensile tails. Arguably, gliding animals prosper in Southeast Asia because the forests are more open (with more room to glide) than those in South America. In dense forests, a prehensile tail enables better tree to tree movement. Also, South American rainforests tend to have more as there are fewer large animals to eat them compared to Africa and Asia; these lianas

Because small animals necessarily have higher surface to volume ratios than larger species of similar form, aerodynamic forces have a greater effect on them, resulting in much lower terminal velocity in free fall and amplifying the effects of even small alterations to body surface area. These small changes provide incremental benefits towards further development of gliding.

Powered Flight

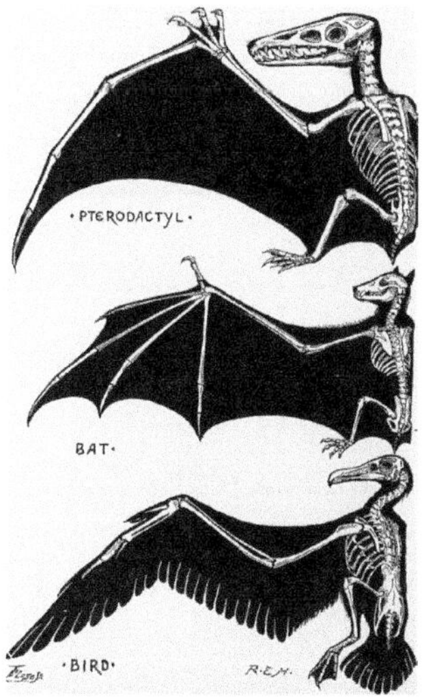

Analogous flying adaptions in vertebrates:
1. pterosaur (Pterosauria) 2. bat (Chiroptera) 3. bird (Aves).

Powered flight has evolved unambiguously only four times—birds, bats, pterosaurs, and insects. In contrast to gliding, which has evolved more frequently but typically gives rise to only a handful of species, all three extant groups of powered flyers have a huge number of species, suggesting that flight is a very successful strategy once evolved. Bats, after rodents, have the most species of any mammalian order, about 20% of all mammalian species. Birds have the most species of any class of terrestrial vertebrates. Finally, insects (most of which fly at some point in their life cycle) have more species than all other animal groups combined.

The evolution of flight is one of the most striking and demanding in animal evolution, and has attracted the attention of many prominent scientists and generated many theories. Additionally, because flying animals tend to be small and have a low mass (both of which increase the surface area to mass ratio), they tend to fossilize infrequently and poorly compared to the larger, heavier-boned terrestrial species they share habitat with. Fossils of flying animals tend to be confined to exceptional fossil deposits formed under highly specific circumstances, resulting in a generally poor fossil record, and a particular lack of transitional forms. Furthermore, as fossils do not preserve behavior or muscle, it can be difficult to discriminate between a poor flyer and a good glider.

Insects were the first to evolve flight, approximately 350 million years ago. The developmental origin of the insect wing remains in dispute, as does the purpose prior to true flight. One suggestion is that wings initially were used to catch the wind for small insects that live on the surface of the water, while another is that they functioned in parachuting, then gliding, then flight for originally arboreal insects.

Pterosaurs were the next to evolve flight, approximately 200 million years ago. These reptiles were close relatives of the dinosaurs (and sometimes mistakenly considered dinosaurs by laymen), and reached enormous sizes, with some of the last forms being the largest flying animals ever to inhabit the Earth, having wingspans of over 9.1 m (30 ft). However, they spanned a large range of sizes, down to a 250 mm (10 in) wingspan in *Nemicolopterus*.

Birds have an extensive fossil record, along with many forms documenting both their evolution from small theropod dinosaurs and the numerous bird-like forms of theropod which did not survive the mass extinction at the end of the Cretaceous. Indeed, *Archaeopteryx* is arguably the most famous transitional fossil in the world, both due to its mix of reptilian and avian anatomy and the luck of being discovered only two years after Darwin's publication of *On the Origin of Species*. However, the ecology and this transition is considerably more contentious, with various scientists supporting either a "trees down" origin (in which an arboreal ancestor evolved gliding, then flight) or a "ground up" origin (in which a fast-running terrestrial ancestor used wings for a speed boost and to help catch prey).

Bats are the most recent to evolve (about 60 million years ago), most likely from a gliding ancestor, though their poor fossil record has hindered more detailed study.

Only a few animals are known to have specialised in soaring: the larger of the extinct pterosaurs, and some large birds. Powered flight is very energetically expensive for large animals, but for soaring their size is an advantage, as it allows them a low wing loading, that is a large wing areas relative to their weight, which maximizes lift. Soaring is very energetically efficient.

Biomechanics

Gliding and Parachuting

During a free-fall with no aerodynamic forces, the object accelerates due to gravity, resulting in increasing velocity as the object descends. During parachuting, animals use the aerodynamic forces on their body to counteract the force or gravity. Any object moving through air experiences a drag force that is proportion to surface area and to velocity squared, and this force will partially counter the force of gravity, slowing the animal's descent to a safer speed. If this drag is oriented at an angle to the vertical, the animal's trajectory will gradually become more horizontal, and it will cover horizontal as well as vertical distance. Smaller adjustments can allow turning or other maneuvers. This can allow a parachuting animal to move from a high location on one tree to a lower location on another tree nearby.

During gliding, lift plays an increased role. Like drag, lift is proportional to velocity squared. Gliding animals will typically leap or drop from high locations such as trees, just as in parachuting, and as gravitational acceleration increases their speed, the aerodynamic forces also increase. Because the animal can utilize lift and drag to generate greater aerodynamic force, it can glide at a shallower angle than parachuting animals, allowing it to cover greater horizontal distance in the same loss of altitude, and reach trees further away.

Powered Flight

Unlike most air vehicles, in which the objects that generate lift (wings) and thrust (engine/propeller) are separate and the wings remained fixed, flying animals use their wings to generate both lift and thrust by moving them relative to the body. This has made the flight of organisms considerably harder to understand than that of vehicles, as it involves varying speeds, angles, orientations, areas, and flow patterns over the wings.

A bird or bat flying through the air at a constant speed moves its wings up and down (usually with some fore-aft movement as well). Because the animal is in motion, there is some airflow relative to its body which, combined with the velocity of with wings, generates a faster airflow moving over the wing. This will generate lift force vector pointing forwards and upwards, and a drag force vector pointing rearwards and upwards. The upwards components of these counteract gravity, keeping the body in the air, while the forward component provides thrust to counteract both the drag from the wing and from the body as a whole. Pterosaur flight likely worked in a similar manner, though no living pterosaurs remain for study.

Insect flight is considerably different, due to their small size, rigid wings, and other anatomical differences. Turbulence and vortices play a much larger role in insect flight, making it even more complex and difficult to study than the flight of vertebrates. There are two basic aerodynamic models of insect flight. Most insects use a method that creates a spiralling leading edge vortex. Some very small insects use the fling-and-clap or Weis-Fogh mechanism in which the wings clap together above the insect's body and then fling apart. As they fling open, the air gets sucked in and creates a vortex over each wing. This bound vortex then moves across the wing and, in the clap, acts as the starting vortex for the other wing. Circulation and lift are increased, at the price of wear and tear on the wings.

Limits and Extremes

Flying/Soaring

- Largest. The largest known flying animal was formerly thought to be *Pteranodon*, a pterosaur with a wingspan of up to 7.5 metres (25 ft). However, the more recently discovered azhdarchid pterosaur *Quetzalcoatlus* is much larger, with estimates of the wingspan ranging from 9 to 12 metres (30 to 39 ft). Some other recently discovered azhdarchid pterosaur species, such as *Hatzegopteryx*, may have also wingspans of a similar size or even slightly larger. Although it is widely thought that *Quetzalcoatlus* reached the size limit of a flying animal, it should be noted that the same was once said of *Pteranodon*. The heaviest living flying animals are the kori bustard and the great bustard with males reaching 21 kilograms (46 lb). The wandering albatross has the greatest wingspan of any living flying animal at 3.63 metres (11.9 ft). Among living animals which fly over land, the Andean condor and the marabou stork have the largest wingspan at 3.2 metres (10 ft). Studies have shown that it is physically possible for flying animals to reach 18-metre (59 ft) wingspans, but there is no firm evidence that any flying animal, not even the azhdarchid pterosaurs, got that large.

- Smallest. There is no real minimum size for getting airborne. Indeed, there are many bacteria floating in the atmosphere that constitute part of the aeroplankton. However, to move about under one's own power and not be overly affected by the wind requires a certain amount of size. The smallest flying vertebrates are the bee hummingbird and the bumblebee bat, both of which may weigh less than 2 grams (0.071 oz). They are thought to represent the lower size limit for endotherm flight.

- Fastest. The fastest of all known flying animals is the peregrine falcon, which when diving travels at 300 kilometres per hour (190 mph) or faster. The fastest animal in flapping horizontal flight may be the Mexican free-tailed bat, said to attain about 160 kilometres per hour (99 mph) based on ground speed by an aircraft tracking device; that measurement does not separate any contribution from wind speed, so the observations could be caused by strong tailwinds.

- Slowest. Most flying animals need to travel forward to stay aloft. However, some creatures can stay in the same spot, known as hovering, either by rapidly flapping the wings, as do hummingbirds, hoverflies, dragonflies, and some others, or carefully using thermals, as do some birds of prey. The slowest flying non-hovering bird recorded is the American woodcock, at 8 kilometres per hour (5.0 mph).

- Highest flying. There are records of a Rüppell's vulture *Gyps rueppelli*, a large vulture, being sucked into a jet engine 11,550 metres (37,890 ft) above Côte d'Ivoire in West Africa. The animal that flies highest most regularly is the bar-headed goose *Anser indicus*, which migrates directly over the Himalayas between its nesting grounds in Tibet and its winter quarters in India. They are sometimes seen flying well above the peak of Mount Everest at 8,848 metres (29,029 ft).

Gliding/parachuting

- Most efficient glider. This can be taken as the animal that moves most horizontal distance per metre fallen. Flying squirrels are known to glide up to 200 metres (660 ft), but have measured glide ratio of about 2. Flying fish have been observed to glide for hundreds of metres on the drafts on the edge of waves with only their initial leap from the water to provide height, but may be obtaining additional lift from wave motion. On the other hand, Albatrosses have measured lift/drag ratios of 20, and thus fall just 1 meter (foot) for every 20 in still air.
- Most maneuverable glider. Many gliding animals have some ability to turn, but which is the most maneuverable is difficult to assess. Even Paradise tree snakes, Chinese gliding frogs, and gliding ants have been observed as having considerable capacity to turn in the air.

Extant Flying and Gliding Animals

Arthropods

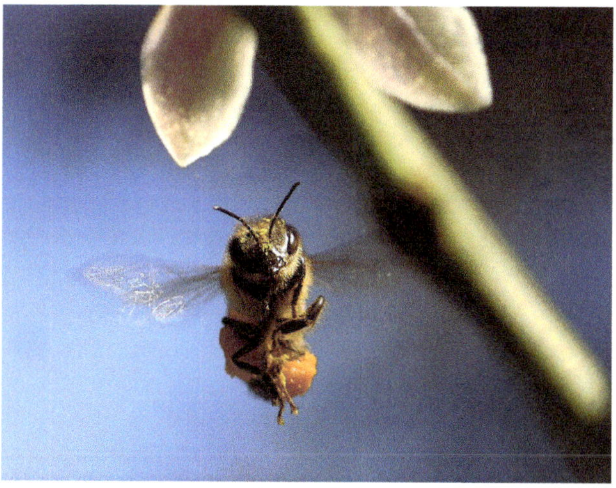

A bee in flight

- Insects (flying). The first of all animals to evolve flight, insects are also the only invertebrates that have evolved flight. The species are too numerous to list here. Insect flight is an active research field.
    - Gliding bristletails (gliding). Directed aerial gliding descent is found in some tropical arboreal bristletails, an ancestrally wingless sister taxa to the winged insects. The bristletails median caudal filament is important for the glide ratio and gliding control

- Gliding ants (gliding). The flightless workers of these insects have secondarily gained some capacity to move through the air. Gliding has evolved independently in a number of arboreal ant species from the groups Cephalotini, Pseudomyrmecinae, and Formicinae (mostly *Camponotus*). All arboreal dolichoderines and non-cephalotine myrmicines except *Daceton armigerum* do not glide. Living in the rainforest canopy like many other gliders, gliding ants use their gliding to return to the trunk of the tree they live on should they fall or be knocked off a branch. Gliding was first discovered for *Cephalotes atreus* in the Peruvian rainforest. *Cephalotes atreus* can make 180 degree turns, and locate the trunk using visual cues, succeeding in landing 80% of the time. Unique among gliding animals, Cephalotini and Pseudomyrmecinae ants glide abdomen first, the Forminicae however glide in the more conventional head first manner. The following page has some good videos of gliding ants.

- Gliding immature insects. The wingless immature stages of some insect species that have wings as adults may also show a capacity to glide. These include some species of cockroach, mantid, katydid, stick insect and true bug.

- Spiders. Although typically flightless some may engage in aerial locomotion as described below.

  - Ballooning spiders (parachuting). The young of some species of spiders travel through the air by using silk draglines to catch the wind, as may some smaller species of adult spider, such the money spider family. This behavior is commonly known as "ballooning". Ballooning spiders make up part of the aeroplankton.

  - Gliding spiders (gliding). Some species of arboreal spider of the genus *Selenops* can glide back to the trunk of a tree should they fall.

Molluscs

- Flying squid (gliding). Several oceanic squids, such as the Pacific flying squid, will leap out of the water to escape predators, an adaptation similar to that of flying fish. Smaller squids will fly in shoals, and have been observed to cover distances as long as 50 metres (160 ft). Small fins towards the back of the mantle do not produce much lift, but do help stabilize the motion of flight. They exit the water by expelling water out of their funnel, indeed some squid have been observed to continue jetting water while airborne providing thrust even after leaving the water. This may make flying squid the only animals with jet-propelled aerial locomotion. The neon flying squid has been observed to glide for distances over 30 metres (100 ft), at speeds of up to 11.2 metres per second (37 ft/s) .

Vertebrates

Fish

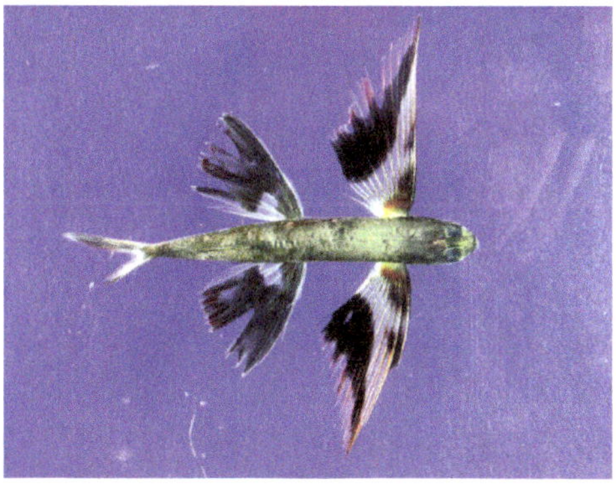

Band-winged flying fish, with enlarged pectoral fins

- Flying fish (gliding). There are over 50 species of flying fish belonging to the family Exocoetidae. They are mostly marine fishes of small to medium size. The largest flying fish can reach lengths of 45 centimetres (18 in) but most species measure less than 30 cm (12 in) in length. They can be divided into two-winged varieties and four-winged varieties. Before the fish leaves the water it increases its speed to around 30 body lengths per second and as it breaks the surface and is freed from the drag of the water it can be traveling at around 60 kilometres per hour (37 mph). The glides are usually up to 30–50 metres (100–160 ft) in length, but some have been observed soaring for hundreds of metres using the updraft on the leading edges of waves. The fish can also make a series of glides, each time dipping the tail into the water to produce forward thrust. The longest recorded series of glides, with the fish only periodically dipping its tail in the water, was for 45 seconds (Video here). It has been suggested that the genus *Exocoetus* is on an evolutionary borderline between flight and gliding. It flaps its enlarged pectoral fins when airborne, but still seems only to glide, as there is no hint of a power stroke. It has been found that some flying fish can glide as effectively as some flying birds.
- Halfbeaks (gliding). A group related to the Exocoetidae, one or two hemirhamphid species possess enlarged pectoral fins and show true gliding flight rather than simple leaps. Marshall (1965) reports that *Euleptorhamphus viridis* can cover 50 metres (160 ft) in two separate hops.
- Freshwater butterflyfish (possibly gliding). *Pantodon buchholzi* has the ability to jump and possibly glide a short distance. It can move through the air several times the length of its body. While it does this, the fish flaps its large pectoral fins, giving it its common name. However, it is debated whether the freshwater butterfly fish can truly glide, Saidel et al. (2004) argue that it cannot.
- Freshwater hatchetfish (possibly flying). There are 9 species of freshwater hatchetfish split among 3 genera. Freshwater hatchetfish have an extremely large sternal

region that is fitted with a large amount of muscle that allows it to flap its pectoral fins. They can move in a straight line over a few metres to escape predators.

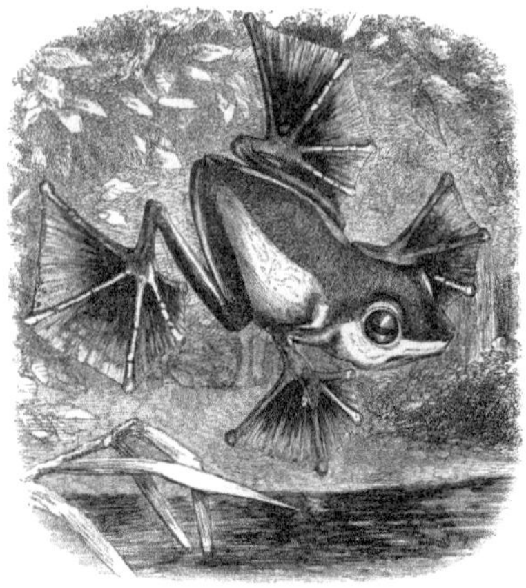

Illustration of Wallace's flying frog in Alfred Russel Wallace's 1869 book *The Malay Archipelago*.

Amphibians

Gliding has evolved independently in two families of tree frogs, the Old World Rhacophoridae and the New World Hylidae. Within each lineage there are a range of gliding abilities from non-gliding, to parachuting, to full gliding.

- Rhacophoridae flying frogs (gliding). A number of the Rhacophoridae, such as Wallace's flying frog (*Rhacophorus nigropalmatus*), have adaptations for gliding, the main feature being enlarged toe membranes. For example, the Malayan flying frog *Rhacophorus prominanus* glides using the membranes between the toes of its limbs, and small membranes located at the heel, the base of the leg, and the forearm. Some of the frogs are quite accomplished gliders, for example, the Chinese flying frog *Rhacophorus dennysi* can maneuver in the air, making two kinds of turn, either rolling into the turn (a banked turn) or yawing into the turn (a crabbed turn).
- Hylidae flying frogs (gliding). The other frog family that contains gliders.

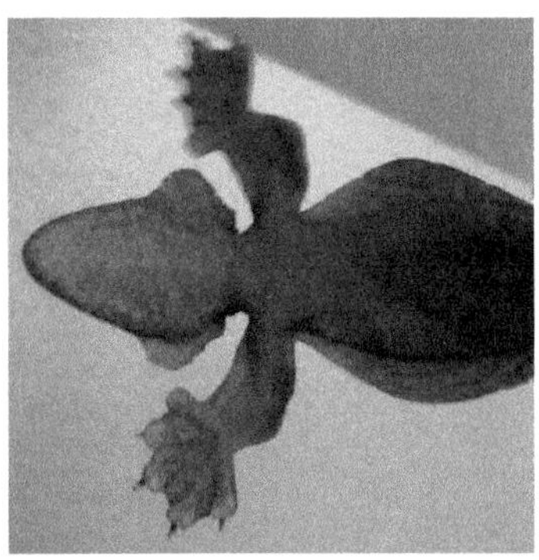

The underside of Kuhl's flying gecko *Ptychozoon kuhli*. The gliding adaptations: flaps of skin on the legs, feet, sides of the body, and on the sides of the head.

Reptiles

Several lizards and snakes are capable of gliding:

- *Draco* lizards. There are 28 species of lizard of the genus *Draco*, found in Sri Lanka, India, and Southeast Asia. They live in trees, feeding on tree ants, but nest on the forest floor. They can glide for up to 60 metres (200 ft) and over this distance they lose only 10 metres (30 ft) in height. Unusually, their patagium (gliding membrane) is supported on elongated ribs rather than the more common situation among gliding vertebrates of having the patagium attached to the limbs. When extended, the ribs form a semicircle on either side the lizard's body and can be folded to the body like a folding fan.
- Gliding lacertids. There are two species of gliding lacertid, of the genus *Holaspis*, found in Africa. They have fringed toes and tail sides and can flatten their bodies for gliding/parachuting.
- *Ptychozoon* flying geckos. There are six species of gliding gecko, of the genus *Ptychozoon*, from Southeast Asia. These lizards have small flaps of skin along their limbs, torso, tail, and head that catch the air and enable them to glide.
- *Lupersaurus* flying geckos. A possible sister-taxon to *Ptychozoon* which has similar flaps and folds and also glides.
- *Thecadactylus* flying geckos. At least some species of *Thecadactylus*, such as *T. rapicauda*, are known to glide.
- *Cosymbotus* flying gecko. Similar adaptations to *Ptychozoon* are found in the two species of the gecko genus *Cosymbotus*.
- *Chrysopelea* snakes. Five species of snake from Southeast Asia, Melanesia, and India. The paradise tree snake of southern Thailand, Malaysia, Borneo, Philippines, and Sulawesi is the most capable glider of those snakes studied. It glides by stretching out its body sideways and opening its ribs so the belly is concave, and by making lateral slithering movements. It can remarkably glide up to 100 metres (330 ft) and make 90 degree turns.

Birds

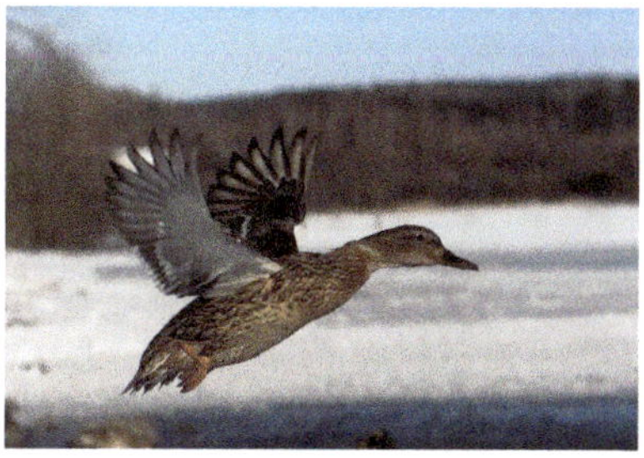

Birds are a successful group of flying vertebrate

- Birds (flying, soaring) — Most of the approximately 10,000 living species can fly (flightless birds are the exception). Bird flight is one of the most studied forms of aerial locomotion in animals.

Mammals

Bats are the only mammal with flapping or powered flight. A few other mammals glide or parachute; the best known are flying squirrels and flying lemurs.

- Bats (flying). There are approximately 1,240 bat species, representing about 20% of all classified mammal species.
- Flying squirrels (subfamily Petauristinae) (gliding). There are 43 species divided between 14 genera of flying squirrel. Flying squirrels are found almost worldwide in tropical (Southeast Asia, India, and Sri Lanka), temperate, and even Arctic environments. They tend to be nocturnal. When a flying squirrel wishes to cross to a tree that is further away than the distance possible by jumping, it extends the cartilage spur on its elbow or wrist. This opens out the flap of furry skin (the patagium) that stretches from its wrist to its ankle. It glides spread-eagle and with its tail fluffed out like a parachute, and grips the tree with its claws when it lands. Flying squirrels have been reported to glide over 200 metres (660 ft).
- Anomalures or scaly-tailed flying squirrels (family Anomaluridae) (gliding). These brightly coloured African rodents are not squirrels but have evolved to a resemble flying squirrels by convergent evolution. There are seven species, divided in three genera. All but one species have gliding membranes between their front and hind legs. The genus *Idiurus* contains two particularly small species known as flying mice, but similarly they are not true mice.
- Colugos or "flying lemurs" (order Dermoptera) (gliding). There are two species of colugo. Despite their common name, colugos are not lemurs; true lemurs are primates. Molecular evidence suggests that colugos are a sister group to primates; however, some mammalogists suggest they are a sister group to bats. Found in Southeast Asia, the colugo is probably the mammal most adapted for gliding, with a patagium that is as large as geometrically possible. They can glide as far as 70 metres (230 ft) with minimal loss of height.
- Sifaka, a type of lemur, and possibly some other primates (possible limited gliding/parachuting). A number of primates have been suggested to have adaptations that allow limited gliding and/or parachuting: sifakas, indris, galagos and saki monkeys. Most notably, the sifaka, a type of lemur, has thick hairs on its forearms that have been argued to provide drag, and a small membrane under its arms that has been suggested to provide lift by having aerofoil properties.

- Flying phalangers or wrist-winged gliders (subfamily Petaurinae) (gliding). Possums found in Australia, and New Guinea. The gliding membranes are hardly noticeable until they jump. On jumping, the animal extends all four legs and stretches the loose folds of skin. The subfamily contains seven species. Of the six species in the genus *Petaurus*, the sugar glider and the Biak glider are the most common species. The lone species in the genus *Gymnobelideus*, Leadbeater's possum has only a vestigial gliding membrane.

- Greater glider (*Petauroides volans*) (gliding). The only species of the genus *Petauroides* of the family Pseudocheiridae. This marsupial is found in Australia, and was originally classed with the flying phalangers, but is now recognised as separate. Its flying membrane only extends to the elbow, rather than to the wrist as in Petaurinae.

- Feather-tailed possums (family Acrobatidae) (gliding). This family of marsupials contains two genera, each with one species. The feathertail glider (*Acrobates pygmaeus*), found in Australia is the size of a very small mouse and is the smallest mammalian glider. The feathertail possum (*Distoechurus pennatus*) is found in New Guinea, but does not glide. Both species have a stiff-haired feather-like tail.

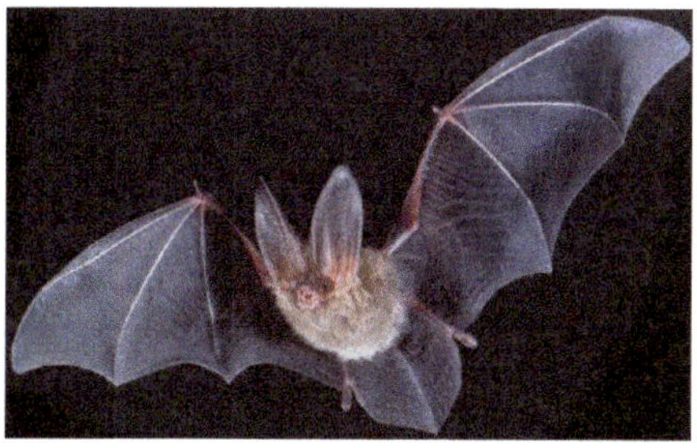

Townsends's big-eared bat, (*Corynorhinus townsendii*) displaying the "hand wing".

Extinct Flying and Gliding Animals

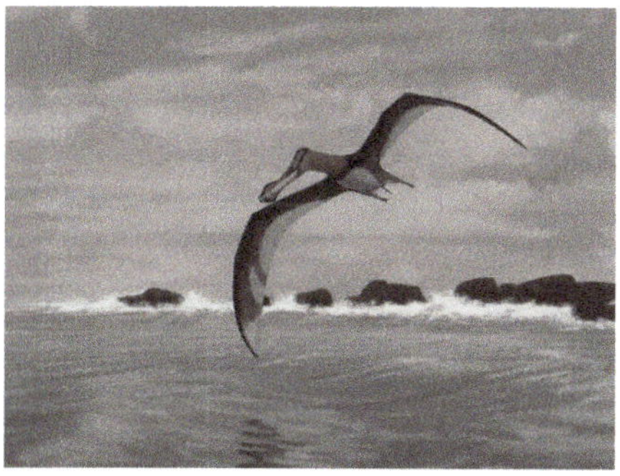

Pterosaurs included the largest known flying animals

Reptiles

- Extinct reptiles similar to *Draco* (gliding). There are a number of unrelated extinct lizard-like reptiles with similar "wings" to the *Draco* lizards. *Icarosaurus, Coelurosauravus, Weigeltisaurus, Mecistotrachelos,* and *Kuehneosaurus.* The largest of these, *Kuehneosaurus,* has a wingspan of 30 centimetres (12 in), and was estimated to be able to glide about 30 metres (100 ft).

- Sharovipterygidae (gliding). These strange reptiles from the Upper Triassic of Kyrgyzstan and Poland unusually had a membrane on their elongated hind limbs, extending their otherwise normal, flying-squirrel-like patagia significantly. The forelimbs are in contrast much smaller.
- *Longisquama insignis* (possibly gliding/parachuting). This small reptile may have had long paired feather-like scales on its back, however it has been more recently argued that the scales form just a single dorsal frill. If paired, they may have been used for parachuting. "Everything you can make out is consistent with it being a small, tree-living, gliding animal, which is precisely the thing you'd expect birds to evolve out of," says Larry Martin, senior curator at the Natural History Museum at the University of Kansas.
- Pterosaurs (flying). Pterosaurs were the first flying vertebrates, and are generally agreed to have been sophisticated flyers. They had large wings formed by a patagium stretching from the torso to a dramatically lengthened fourth finger. There were hundreds of species, most of which are thought to have been intermittent flappers, and many soarers. The largest known flying animals are pterosaurs.
- *Hypuronector* (gliding). This bizarre drepanosaur displays limb proportions, particularly the elongated forelimbs, that are consistent with a flying or gliding animal with patagia.

Non-avian Dinosaurs

- Theropods (gliding/flying). There were several species of theropod dinosaur thought to be capable of gliding or flying, that are not classified as birds (though they are closely related). Some species (*Microraptor gui, Microraptor zhaoianus, Cryptovolans pauli,* and *Changyuraptor*) have been found that were fully feathered on all four limbs, giving them four 'wings' that they are believed to have used for gliding or flying. One species, *Deinonychus antirrhopus,* may display partial volancy, with the young being capable of flight while the adults are flightless, a characteristic also seen in some modern birds like the Horned coot and the Flying steamer duck.
- *Yi* is unique among gliding dinosaurs for the development of membranous wings, unlike the feathered airfoils of other theropods. Much like modern anomalures it developed a bony rod to help support the wing, albeit on the wrist and not the elbow.

Fish

- Thoracopteridae (gliding) is a lineage of Triassic flying fish-like Perleidiformes, having converted their pectoral and pelvic fins into broad wings very similar to those of their modern counterparts. The Ladinian genus *Potanichthys* is the oldest member of this clade, as well as the earliest aerial vertebrate known, suggesting that these fish began exploring aerial niches soon after the Permian-Triassic extinction event.

Mammals

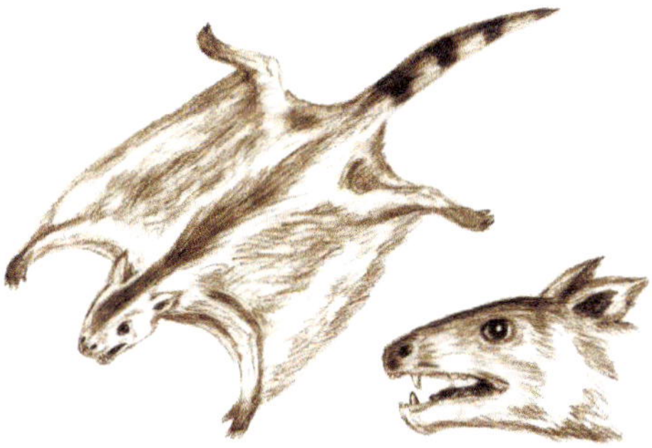

Volaticotherids predate bats as mammalian aeronauts by at least 110 million years.

- *Volaticotherium antiquum* (gliding). The earliest known flying or gliding mammal. This squirrel-sized animal belonged to a now extinct ancestral line and was not related to modern day flying or gliding mammals, such as bats or gliding marsupials. It lived around 164 million years ago and used a fur-covered skin membrane to glide through the air. The closely related *Argentoconodon* is also thought to have been able to glide, based on postcranial similarities; it lived around 165 million years ago.
- Several species of extinct bat have been found, like *Icaronycteris*, *Palaeochiropteryx*, and *Onychonycteris*.
- A gliding metatherian (possibly a marsupial) is known from the Paleocene of Itaboraí, Brazil.

Terrestrial Locomotion

Terrestrial locomotion has evolved as animals adapted from aquatic to terrestrial environments. Locomotion on land raises different problems than that in water, with reduced friction being replaced by the effects of gravity.

There are three basic forms of locomotion found among terrestrial animals

- Legged - Moving by using appendages

- Limbless locomotion - moving without legs, primarily using the body itself as a propulsive structure.
- Rolling - rotating the body over the substrate

Legged Locomotion

Movement on appendages is the most common form of terrestrial locomotion, it is the basic form of locomotion of two major groups with many terrestrial members, the vertebrates and the arthropods. Important aspects of legged locomotion are posture (the way the body is supported by the legs), the number of legs, and the functional structure of the leg and foot. There are also many gaits, ways of moving the legs to locomote, such as walking, running, or jumping.

Posture

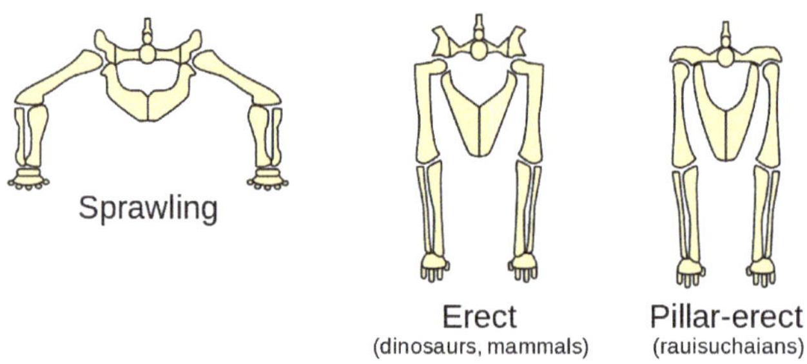

Hip joints and hindlimb postures

Appendages can be used for movement in a number of ways. The posture, the way the body is supported by the legs, is an important aspect. There are three main ways in which vertebrates support themselves with their legs - sprawling, semi-erect, and fully erect. Some animals may use different postures in different circumstances, depending on the posture's mechanical advantages. Interestingly, there is no detectable difference in energetic cost between stances.

The "sprawling" posture is the most primitive, and is the original limb posture from which the others evolved. The upper limbs are typically held horizontally, while the lower limbs are vertical, though upper limb angle may be substantially increased in large animals. The body may drag along the ground, as in salamanders, or may be substantially elevated, as in monitor lizards. This posture is typically associated with trotting gaits, and the body flexes from side-to-side during movement to increase step length. All limbed reptiles and salamanders use this posture, as does the platypus and several species of frogs that walk. Unusual examples can be found among amphibious fish, such as the mudskipper, which drag themselves across land on their sturdy fins. Among the invertebrates, most arthropods—which includes the most diverse group of animals, the insects—have a stance best described as sprawling. There is also anecdotal evidence that some octopus species (such as the *Pinnoctopus* genus) can also drag themselves across land a short distance by hauling their body along by their tentacles (for example to pursue prey between rockpools) - there may be video evidence of this. The semi-erect posture is more accurately interpreted as an extremely elevated sprawling posture. This mode of locomotion is typically found in large lizards such as monitor lizards and tegus.

Mammals and birds typically have a fully erect posture, though each evolved it independently. In these groups the legs are placed beneath the body. This is often linked with the evolution of endothermy, as it avoids Carrier's constraint and thus allows prolonged periods of activity. The fully erect stance is not necessarily the "most-evolved" stance; evidence suggests that crocodilians evolved a semi-erect stance in their forelimbs from ancestors with fully erect stance as a result of adapting to a mostly aquatic lifestyle, though their hindlimbs are still held fully erect. For example, the mesozoic prehistoric crocodilian *Erpetosuchus* is believed to have had a fully erect stance and been terrestrial.

Number of Legs

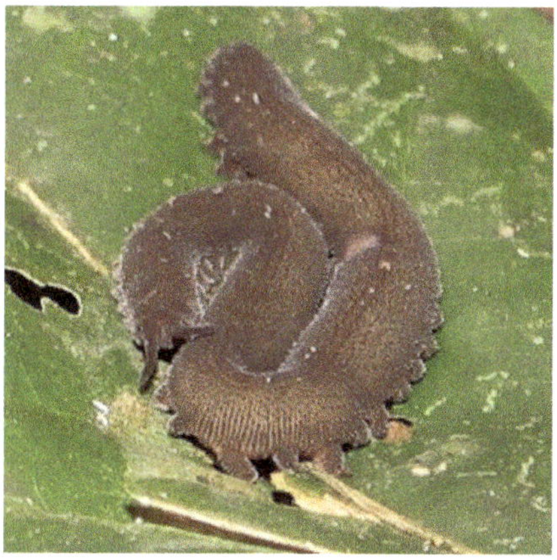

The velvet worm (Onychophora)

The number of locomotory appendages varies much between animals, and sometimes the same animal may use different numbers of its legs in different circumstances. The best contender for unipedal movement is the springtail, which while normally hexapedal, hurls itself away from danger using its furcula, a tail-like forked rod that can be rapidly unfurled from the underside of its body.

A number of species move and stand on two legs, that is, they are bipedal. The group that is exclusively bipedal is the birds, which have either an alternating or a hopping gait. There are also a number of bipedal mammals. Most of these move by hopping – including the macropods such as kangaroos and various jumping rodents. Only a few mammals such as humans and the ground pangolin commonly show an alternating bipedal gait. Cockroaches and some lizards may also run on their two hind legs.

With the exception of the birds, terrestrial vertebrate groups with legs are mostly quadrupedal – the mammals, reptiles, and the amphibians usually move on four legs. There are many quadrupedal gaits. The most diverse group of animals on earth, the insects, are included in a larger taxon known as hexapods, most of which are hexapedal, walking and standing on six legs. Exceptions among the insects include praying mantises and water scorpions, which are quadrupeds with their front two legs modified for grasping, some butterflies such as the Lycaenidae (blues and hairstreaks) which use only four legs, and some kinds of insect larvae that may have no legs (e.g., maggots), or additional prolegs (e.g., caterpillars).

Spiders and many of their relatives move on eight legs – they are octopedal. However, some creatures move on many more legs. Terrestrial crustaceans may have a fair number - woodlice having fourteen legs. Also, as previously mentioned, some insect larvae such as caterpillars and sawfly larvae have up to five (caterpillars) or nine (sawflies) additional fleshy prolegs in addition to the six legs normal for insects. Some species of invertebrate have even more legs, the unusual velvet worm having stubby legs under the length of its body, with around several dozen pairs of legs. Centipedes have one pair of legs per body segment, with typically around 50 legs, but some species have over 200. The terrestrial animals with the most legs are the millipedes. They have two pairs of legs per body segment, with common species having between 80 and 400 legs overall – with the rare species *Illacme plenipes* having up to 750 legs. Animals with many legs typically move them in metachronal rhythm, which gives the appearance of waves of motion travelling forwards along their rows of legs.

Leg and Foot Structure

The legs of tetrapods, the main group of terrestrial vertebrates, have internal bones, with externally attached muscles for movement, and the basic form has three key joints: the shoulder joint, the knee joint, and the ankle joint, at which the foot is attached. Within this theme there is much variation in form. An alternative form of vertebrate 'leg' to the tetrapod leg is the fins found on amphibious fish. Also a few tetrapods, such as the macropods, have adapted their tails as additional locomotory appendages.

The basic form of the vertebrate foot has five toes, however some animals will have evolved fewer than this, and some early tetrapods had more; Acanthostega had eight toes. Feet have evolved many forms depending on the animal's needs. One key variation is where on the foot the animal's weight is placed. Most vertebrates—the amphibians, the reptiles, and some mammals such as humans and bears—are plantigrade, walking on the whole of the underside of the foot. Many mammals, such as cats and dogs are digitigrade, walking on their toes, the greater stride length allowing more speed. Digitigrade mammals are also often adept at quiet movement. Birds are also digitigrade. Some animals such as horses are unguligrade, walking on the tips of their toes. This even further increases their stride length and thus their speed. A few mammals are also known to walk on their knuckles, at least for their front legs. Knuckle-walking allows the foot (hand) to specialise for food gathering and/or climbing, as with the great apes and the extinct chalicotheres, or for swimming, as with the platypus. In animals where feet have evolved into functional hands, hand walking is also possible.

Among terrestrial invertebrates there are a number of leg forms. The arthropod legs are jointed and supported by hard external armor, with the muscles attached to the internal surface of this exoskeleton. The other group of legged terrestrial invertebrates, the velvet worms, have soft stumpy legs supported by a hydrostatic skeleton. The prolegs that some caterpillars have in addition to their six more-standard arthropod legs have a similar form to those of velvet worms, and suggest a distant shared ancestry.

Gaits

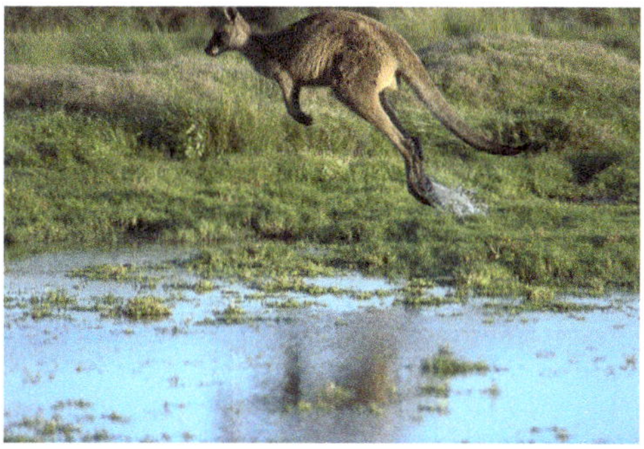

A jumping kangaroo

Animals show a vast range of gaits, the order that they place and lift their appendages in locomotion. Gaits can be grouped into categories according to their patterns of support sequence. For quadrupeds, there are three main categories: walking gaits, running gaits, and leaping gaits. In one system (relating to horses), there are 60 discrete patterns: 37 walking gaits, 14 running gaits, and 9 leaping gaits.

Walking is the most common gait, where some feet are on the ground at any given time, and found in almost all legged animals. In an informal sense, running is considered to occur when at some points in the stride all feet are off the ground in a moment of suspension. Technically, however, moments of suspension occur in both running gaits (such as trot) and leaping gaits (such as canter and gallop). Gaits involving one or more moments of suspension can be found in many animals, and compared to walking they are faster but more energetically costly forms of locomotion.

Animals will use different gaits for different speeds, terrain, and situations. For example, horses show four natural gaits, the slowest horse gait is the walk, then there are three faster gaits which, from slowest to fastest, are the trot, the canter, and the gallop. Animals may also have unusual gaits that are used occasionally, such as for moving sideways or backwards. For example, the main human gaits are bipedal walking and running, but they employ many other gaits occasionally, including a four-legged crawl in tight spaces.

In walking, and for many animals running, the motion of legs on either side of the body alternates, i.e. is out of phase. Other animals, such as a horse when galloping, or an inchworm, alternate between their front and back legs. An alternative to a gait that alternates between legs is hopping or saltation, where all legs move together. As a main means of locomotion, this is usually found in bipeds or semi-bipeds. Among the mammals saltation is commonly used among macropods (kangaroos and their relatives), jerboas, springhares, kangaroo rats, hopping mice, gerbils, and sportive lemurs. Certain tendons in kangaroo hind legs are very elastic, allowing kangaroos to effectively bounce along conserving energy from hop to hop, making hopping a very energy efficient way to move around in their nutrient poor environment. Saltation is also used by many small birds. Frogs and fleas also hop.

Most animals move in the direction of their head. However, there are some exceptions. Crabs move sideways, and naked mole rats, which live in tight tunnels underground, can move backward or forward with equal facility. Crayfish can move backward much faster than they can move forward.

Gait analysis is the study of gait in humans and other animals. This may involve videoing subjects with markers on particular anatomical landmarks and measuring the forces of their footfall using floor transducers (strain gauges). Skin electrodes may also be used to measure muscle activity.

Limbless Locomotion

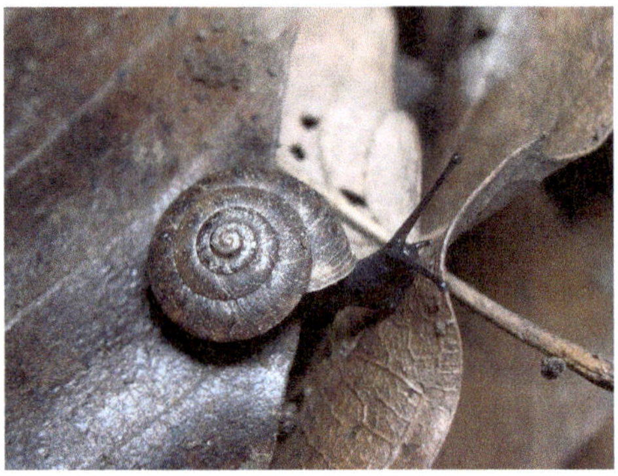

A snail moves by slithering

There are a number of terrestrial and amphibious limbless vertebrates and invertebrates. These animals, due to lack of appendages, use their bodies to generate propulsive force. These movements are sometimes referred to as "slithering" or "crawling", although neither are formally used in the scientific literature and the latter term is also used for some animals moving on all four limbs. All limbless animals come from cold-blooded groups; there are no endothermic limbless animals, i.e. there are no limbless birds or mammals.

Lower Body Surface

Where the foot is important to the legged mammal, for limbless animals the underside of the body is important. Some animals such as snakes or legless lizards move on their smooth dry underside. Other animals have various features that aid movement. Molluscs such as slugs and snails move on a layer of mucus that is secreted from their underside, reducing friction and protecting from injury when moving over sharp objects. Earthworms have small bristles (setae) that hook into the substrate and help them move. Some animals such as leeches have suction cups on either end of the body allowing two anchor movement.

Type of Movement

Some limbless animals, such as leeches, have suction cups on either end of their body, which allow them to move by anchoring the rear end and then moving forward the front end, which is then anchored and then the back end is pulled in, and so on. This is known as two-anchor movement. A legged animal, the inchworm, also moves like this, clasping with appendages at either end of its body.

Limbless animals can also move using pedal locomotary waves, rippling the underside of the body. This is the main method used by molluscs such as slugs and snails, and also large flatworms, some other worms, and even earless seals. The waves may move in the opposite direction to motion, known as retrograde waves, or in the same direction as motion, known as direct waves. Earthworms move by retrograde waves alternatively swelling and contracting down the length of their body, the swollen sections being held in place using setae. Aquatic molluscs such as limpets, which are sometimes out of the water, tend to move using retrograde waves. However terrestrial molluscs such as slugs and snails tend to use direct waves. Lugworms and seals also use direct waves.

Most snakes move using lateral undulation where a lateral wave travels down the snake's body in the opposite direction to the snake's motion and pushes the snake off irregularities in the ground. This mode of locomotion requires these irregularities to function. Another form of locomotion, rectilinear locomotion, is used at times by some snakes, especially large ones such as pythons and boa. Here large scales on the underside of the body, known as scutes are used to push backwards and downwards. This is effective on a flat surface and is used for slow, silent movement, such as when stalking prey. Snakes use concertina locomotion for moving slowly in tunnels, here the snake alternates in bracing parts of its body on it surrounds. Finally the caenophidian snakes use the fast and unusual method of movement known as sidewinding on sand or loose soil. The snake cycles through throwing the front part of its body in the direction of motion and bringing the back part of its body into line crosswise.

Rolling

Although animals have never evolved wheels for locomotion, a small number of animals will move at times by rolling their whole body. Rolling animals can be divided into those that roll under the force of gravity or wind and those that roll using their own power.

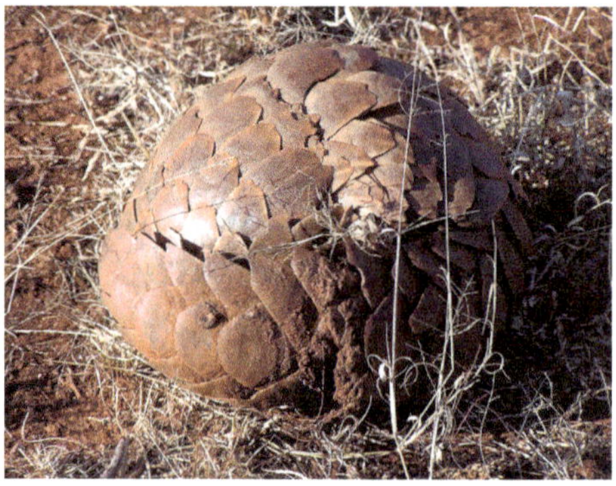

The pangolin *Manis temminckii* in defensive position.

Gravity or Wind Assisted

The web-toed salamander, a 10-centimetre (3.9 in) salamander, lives on steep hills in the Sierra Nevada mountains. When disturbed or startled it coils itself up into a ball, often causing it to roll downhill.

The pebble toad (*Oreophrynella nigra*) lives atop tepui in the Guiana highlands of South America. When threatened, often by tarantulas, it rolls into ball, and typically being on an incline, rolls away under gravity like a loose pebble.

Namib wheeling spiders (*Carparachne spp.*), found in the Namib desert, will actively roll down sand dunes. This action can be used to successfully escape predators such as the *Pompilidae* tarantula wasps, which lay their eggs in a paralyzed spider for their larvae to feed on when they hatch. The spiders flip their body sideways and then cartwheel over their bent legs. The rotation is fast, the golden wheel spider (*Carparachne aureoflava*) moving up to 20 revolutions per second, moving the spider at 1 metre per second.

Coastal tiger beetle larvae when threatened can flick themselves into the air and curl their bodies to form a wheels, which the wind blows, often uphill, as far as 25m and as fast as 11kph. The also may have some ability to steer themselves in this state.

Pangolins, a type of mammal covered in thick scales, roll into a tight ball when threatened. Pangolins have been reported to roll away from danger, by both gravity and self-powered methods. A pangolin in hill country in Sumatra, to flee from the researcher, ran to the edge of a slope and curled into a ball to roll down the slope, crashing through the vegetation, and covering an estimated 30 metres or more in 10 seconds.

Self-powered

Caterpillars of the Mother-Of-Pearl Moth, *Pleuroptya ruralis*, when attacked, will touch their heads to their tails and roll backwards, up to 5 revolutions at about 40 cm per second, which is about 40 times its normal speed.

Nannosquilla decemspinosa, a species of long-bodied, short-legged mantis shrimp, lives in shallow sandy areas along the Pacific coast of Central and South America. When stranded by a low tide the 3 cm stomatopod lies on its back and performs backwards somersaults over and over. The animal moves up to 2 meters at a time by rolling 20–40 times, with speeds of around 72 revolutions per minute. That is 1.5 body lengths per second (3.5 cm/s). Researchers estimate that the stomatopod acts as a true wheel around 40% of the time during this series of rolls. The remaining 60% of the time it has to "jumpstart" a roll by using its body to thrust itself upwards and forwards.

Pangolins have also been reported to roll away from danger by self-powered methods. Witnessed by a lion researcher in the Serengeti in Africa, a group of lions surrounded a pangolin, but could not get purchase on it when it rolled into a ball, and so the lions sat around it waiting and dozing. Surrounded by lions, it would unroll itself slightly and give itself a push to roll some distance, until by doing this multiple times it could get far enough away from the lions to be safe. Moving like this would allow a pangolin to cover distance while still remaining in a protective armoured ball.

Limits and Extremes

The fastest terrestrial animal is the cheetah, which can attain maximal sprint speeds of approximately 104 km/h (64 mph). The fastest running lizard is the Black Iguana, which has been recorded moving at speed of up to 34.9 km/h (21.7 mph).

Trot

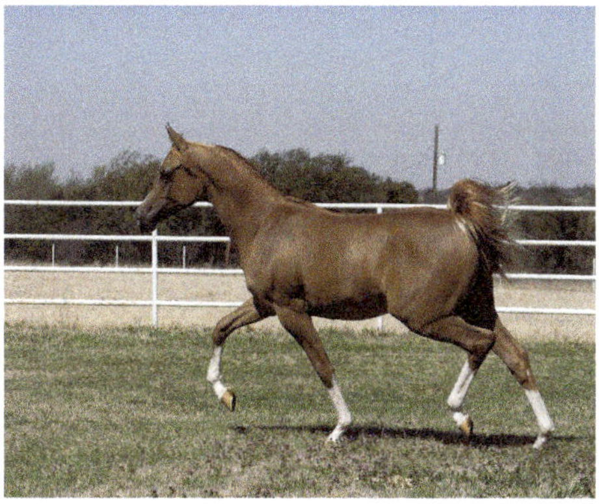

The trot

The trot is a two-beat diagonal gait of the horse where the diagonal pairs of legs move forward at the same time with a moment of suspension between each beat. It has a wide variation in possible speeds, but averages about 8 miles per hour (13 km/h). A very slow trot is sometimes referred to as a jog. An extremely fast trot has no special name, but in harness racing, the trot of a Standardbred is faster than the gallop of the average non-racehorse, and has been clocked at over 30 miles per hour (48 km/h).

June 29, 2014 at Pocono Downs in Pennsylvania the Swedish standardbred Sebastian K ran a mile in 1 minute, 49 seconds (quarters were passed at 26:2, 55:3 and 1,21:4). This is equivalent to a 1000-pace in 1.07,7 or 53,14 kilometers per hour or 33 miles per hour.

From the standpoint of the balance of the horse, the trot is a very stable gait and does not require the horse to make major balancing motions with its head and neck. Due to its many variations, the trot is a common gait that the horse is worked in for dressage.

Eadweard Muybridge was the first to prove, by photography, in 1872 that there is a "moment of suspension" or "unsupported transit" during the trot gait.

Types

Depending on the amount of engagement and collection of the horse, the trot can generally be classified as "working", "collected", or "extended". By the rhythm, one may distinguish a true, two-beat square trot when each diagonal pair of hoofs hits the ground at the same moment from a four-beat intermediate ambling gait, such as the fox trot or the "trocha" sometimes seen in the Paso Fino.

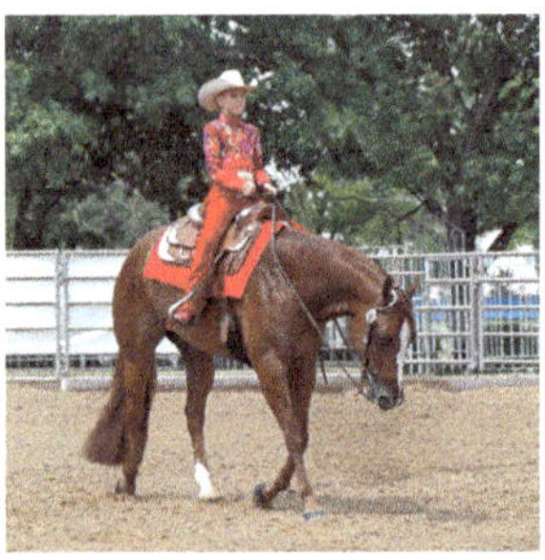

Jog trot

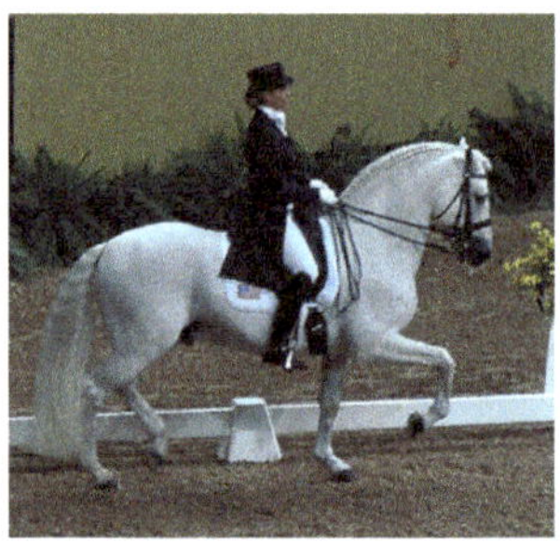

Collected trot

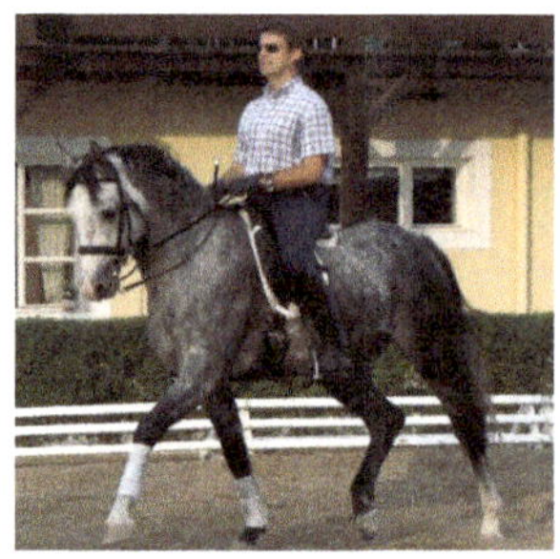

Working trot

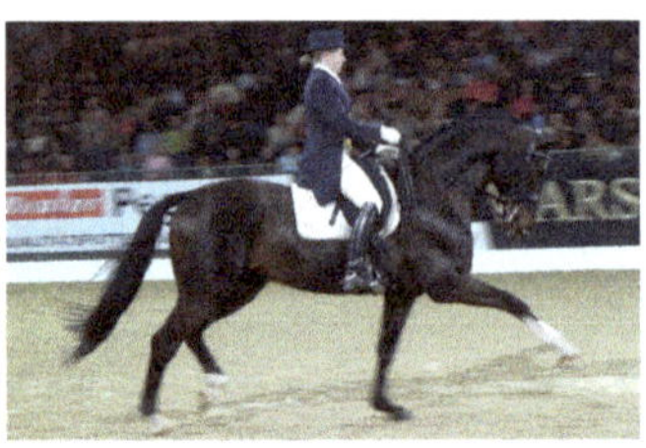

Medium trot

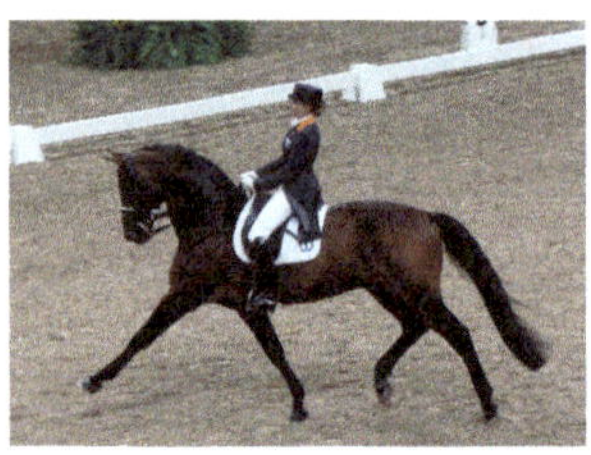

Extended trot

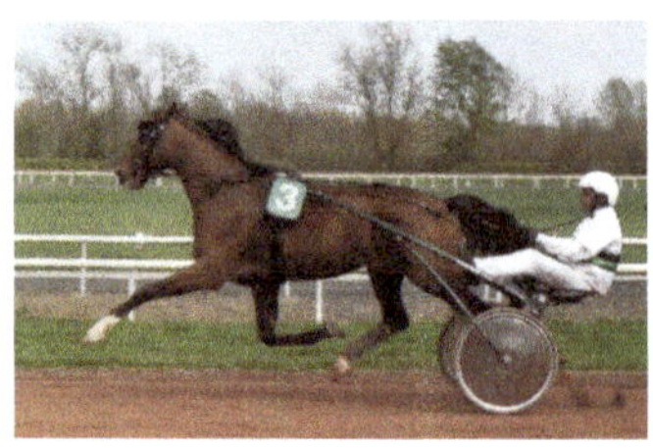

Racing trot

Different speeds and types of trots are described by the following terms:

- Jog trot, as seen in western horses, is a slow, relaxed trot lacking the suspension of a working trot and with shorter strides. It is easy to ride because there is less "bounce". The head of the horse is carried low while the hindquarters are engaged and underneath the horse, and there is less impulsion than in a dressage-style collected trot.

- Collected trot: A very engaged trot where most of the horse's weight is carried toward the hindquarters. The frame is compressed and the stride length is shorter than any of the other trots with the horse taking higher steps. The horse is lighter and more mobile in the collected trot.
- Slow trot (harness) or Road gait (roadster): Is slower than a working trot, but faster than a jog trot. This gait is one of the gaits used in harness classes at horse shows.
- Working trot or Trot: The stride length (some breeds have naturally varied strides) is "normal" for the horse and is the natural trot of the horse when under saddle. It is a gait between the collected trot and medium trot.
- Medium trot: A trot that is more engaged and rounder than the working trot with moderately extended strides and good, solid impulsion. The medium trot lies between the working and the extended trot.
- Park trot: Sometimes simply called a Trot in a given class and seen in saddle seat and fine harness classes for Saddlebreds, Arabians and Morgans. It is a showy, flashy trot with extreme elevation of the knees (forearm is horizontal or higher and the hind legs are extremely flexed). The head is held high and at times a horse may hollow its back and lose cadence in an attempt to achieve high action in front. The hindquarters must be engaged for it to be properly performed.
- Lengthened trot: A trot with lengthened strides. It differs from the more advanced extended trot in that it does not require the horse to bring its weight as far back on its hindquarters.
- Road trot or Show at Speed: As seen in roadster classes, is a gait similar to a racing trot, but much slower (suitable for an arena setting). The horse's head is collected, the stride is at maximum length, and the step is high and animated.
- Extended trot: An engaged trot with long strides where the horse stretches its frame and lengthens its strides to the greatest degree possible. The horse has a great amount of suspension. The back is round and the horse's head just in front and vertical.
- Racing trot: As seen in harness racing horses that race at a trot, such as Standardbred. The stride is at its maximum length with a great deal of suspension. The hind leg in a diagonal pair may begin to hit the ground before the front. Unlike the extended trot, the neck is not round but is extended out. As of September 2013, the North American speed record for a racing trot under saddle at one mile is 1:59, or 30.25 miles per hour (48.68 km/h)

Haute Ecole Variations on the Trot

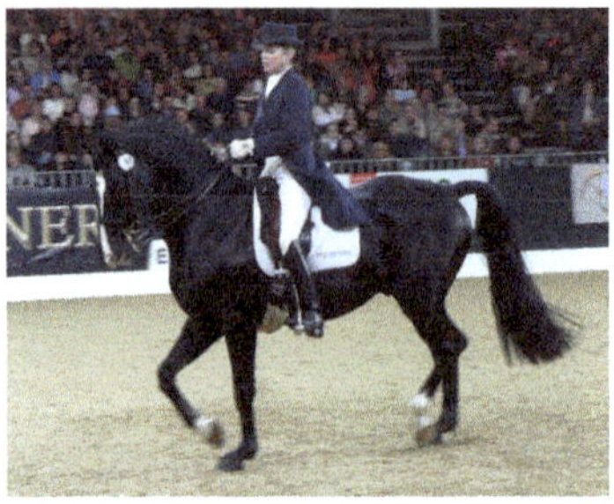

Passage

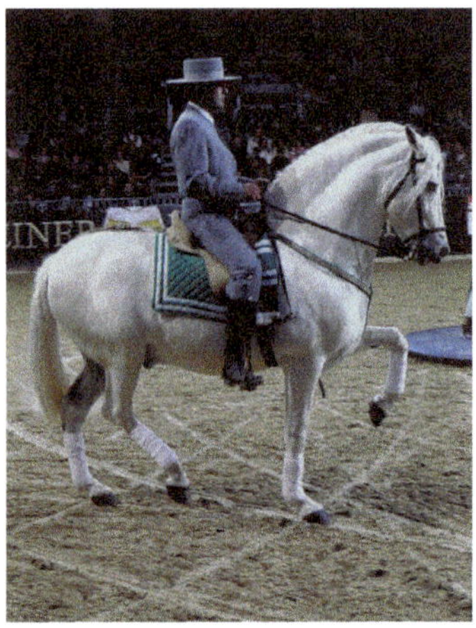

Piaffe

Two variations of the trot are specially trained in advanced dressage horses: the Piaffe and the Passage. The Piaffe is essentially created by asking the horse to trot in place, with very little forward motion. The Passage (rhymes with "massage") is an exaggerated slow motion trot. Both require tremendous collection, careful training and considerable physical conditioning for a horse to perform.

Riding Technique

Depending on the horse and its speed, a trot can be difficult for a rider to sit because the body of the horse actually drops a bit between beats and bounces up again when the next set of legs strike the ground. Each time another diagonal pair of legs hits the ground, the rider can be jolted upwards out of the saddle and meet the horse with some force on the way back down. Therefore, at most speeds above a jog, especially in English riding disciplines, most riders *post* to the trot, rising up and down in rhythm with the horse to avoid being jolted. Posting is easy on the horse's back, and once mastered is also easy on the rider.

To not be jostled out of the saddle and to not harm the horse by bouncing on its back, riders must learn specific skills in order to sit the trot. Most riders learn to sit a slow jog trot without bouncing. A skilled rider can ride a powerfully extended trot without bouncing, but to do so requires well-conditioned back and abdominal muscles, and to do so for long periods is tiring for even experienced riders. A fast, uncollected, racing trot, such as that of the harness racing horse, is virtually impossible to sit.

Because the trot is such a safe and efficient gait for a horse, learning to ride the trot correctly is an important component in almost all equestrian disciplines, particularly for equitation riders. "Gaited" or "ambling" horses, which have smooth 4-beat intermediate gaits that replace or supplement the trot, are popular with riders who prefer for various reasons not to have to ride at a trot.

There are three ways the trot may be ridden:

- Sitting: The rider's seat remains in the saddle the whole time while following the motion of the horse and without bouncing. This is required for show ring western riding and preferred in dressage, especially at the upper levels. Sitting the trot gives the rider optimum control, because he or she can use the seat and weight to ask the horse to make upward or downward transitions, turns, and/or to decrease or increase impulsion. It is also a test of equitation by proving that the rider can quietly move with the horse. The jog, which is the preferred gait of western horses, is generally smoother and less-bouncy than the working and extended trot of the English-style horse. Sitting can be very tiring for the rider, especially if performed by riders who have not built up their stomach and back muscles, or if riders are on an extremely powerful mount with a big trot. To sit the trot, there is a slight forward and back movement of the lower back and stomach as the rider's hips follow both the up and down and side-to-side motion of the horse. To absorb the impact of the trot, the rider relaxes through the hips and the stomach and lower back, as well as the legs. The rider's upper body remains upright and quiet. The rider's hands remain steady. The lower legs remain relaxed and only come into play when the rider gives a leg aid. If a rider cannot sit the trot and is bounced around, the rising trot is preferable, because not only is the rider uncomfortable, the constant slamming of the rider onto the horse is uncomfortable for the horse. As a result, it will hollow its back and stiffen its movement.

- Rising or Posting: The rider makes an up-and-down movement each stride, rising out of the saddle for one beat and lowering (sits) for the second beat. When the rising trot is performed correctly, it is comfortable for the rider and easy on the horse. This is preferred for show jumping, hunt seat, eventing (the jumping phases), saddle seat, lower-level dressage, and most other English-type riding as well as endurance riding. Although this does not provide as much control as sitting, it frees the horse's back. In the rising trot, the rider allows the horse's movement to throw his or her seat a bit out of the saddle. When coming back down, the seat touches down lightly rather than slamming down on the horse's back. Except in saddle seat riding, rider's shoulders maintain a slight forward incline throughout the rising trot, instead of the upright, vertical position seen in sitting trot. The shoulders and lower legs remain in relatively the same position when the rider is both rising and sitting and the hands also stay in the same position as the rider rises and sits.

- Half-seat or Two-point: Also called a jumping position. Sometimes used synonymously, the half-seat variation involves the rider getting the seat bones off the saddle and keeping soft contact with the pelvis, and two-point variation involves the rider raising the seat and pelvic bones. In both cases, the rider remains off the saddle and does not sit or post. This provides a great deal of freedom for the horse's back. It also offers the least amount of control for the rider. These positions are rarely used at the trot; although, both are common at the canter for jumping riders. Two-point position also requires a good amount of strength in the rider's legs.

Diagonals

A rider posts to one "diagonal" or the other at the trot; when the rider is on the correct diagonal, the rider sits as the horse's inside hind leg and outside foreleg are on the ground and rises as the outside hind leg and inside foreleg are on the ground. Diagonals are used in the posting trot help to keep the horse balanced, and are also useful for timing certain riding aids, such as those for the canter. A rider can learn to recognize diagonals by feel. However, less-experienced riders can check for the correct diagonal by a quick glance at the horse's shoulder, sitting when the outside foreleg is on the ground and the is shoulder back.

Undulatory Locomotion

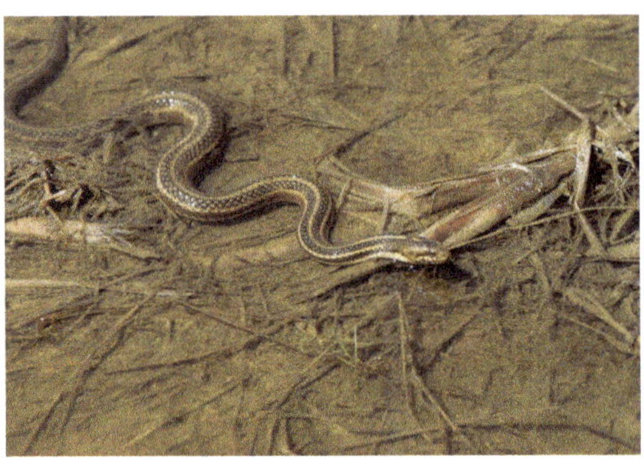

Snakes primarily rely on undulatory locomotion to move through a wide range of environments.

Undulatory locomotion is the type of motion characterized by wave-like movement patterns that act to propel an animal forward. Examples of this type of gait include crawling in snakes, or swimming in the lamprey. Although this is typically the type of gait utilized by limbless animals, some creatures with limbs, such as the salamander, choose to forgo use of their legs in certain environments and exhibit undulatory locomotion. This movement strategy is important to study in order to create novel robotic devices capable of traversing a variety of environments.

Environmental Interactions

In limbless locomotion, forward locomotion is generated by propagating flexural waves along the length of the animal's body. Forces generated between the animal and surrounding environment lead to a generation of alternating sideways forces that act to move the animal forward. These forces generate thrust and drag.

Hydrodynamics

Simulation predicts that thrust and drag are dominated by viscous forces at low Reynolds numbers and inertial forces at higher Reynolds numbers. When the animal swims in a fluid, two main forces are thought to play a role:

- Skin Friction: Generated due to the resistance of a fluid to shearing and is proportional to speed of the flow. This dominates undulatory swimming in spermatozoa and the nematode
- Form Force: Generated by the differences in pressure on the surface of the body and it varies with the square of flow speed.

At low Reynolds number ($Re \sim 10^0$), skin friction accounts for nearly all of the thrust and drag. For those animals which undulate at intermediate Reynolds number ($Re \sim 10^1$), such as the Ascidian larvae, both skin friction and form force account for the production of drag and thrust. At high Reynolds number ($Re \sim 10^2$), both skin friction and form force act to generate drag, but only form force produces thrust.

Kinematics

In animals that move without use of limbs, the most common feature of the locomotion is a rostral to caudal wave that travels down their body. However, this pattern can change based on the particular undulating animal, the environment, and the metric in which the animal is optimizing (i.e. speed, energy, etc.). The most common mode of motion is simple undulations in which lateral bending is propagated from head to tail.

Snakes can exhibit 5 different modes of terrestrial locomotion: (1) lateral undulation, (2) sidewinding, (3) concertina, (4) rectilinear, and (5) slide-pushing. Lateral undulation closely resembles the simple undulatory motion observed in many other animals such as in lizards, eels and fish, in which waves of lateral bending propagate down the snake's body.

The American eel typically moves in an aquatic environment, though it can also move on land for short periods of time. It is able to successfully move about in both environments by producing traveling waves of lateral undulations. However, differences between terrestrial and aquatic locomotor strategy suggest that the axial musculature is being activated differently. In terrestrial locomotion, all points along the body move on approximately the same path and, therefore, the lateral displacements along the length of the eel's body is approximately the same. However, in aquatic locomotion, different points along the body follow different paths with increasing lateral amplitude more posteriorly. In general, the amplitude of the lateral undulation and angle of intervertebral flexion is much greater during terrestrial locomotion than that of aquatic.

Musculoskeletal System

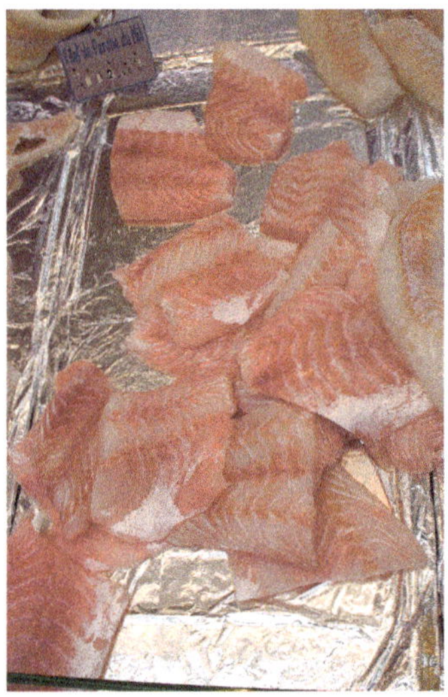

Perch filets showing myomere structure

Muscle Architecture

A typical characteristic of many animals that utilize undulatory locomotion is that they have segmented muscles, or blocks of myomeres, running from their head to tails which are separated by connective tissue called myosepta. In addition, some segmented muscle groups, such as the lateral hypaxial musculature in the salamander are oriented at an angle to the longitudinal direction. For these obliquely oriented fibers the strain in the longitudinal direction is greater than the strain in the muscle fiber direction leading to an architectural gear ratio greater than 1. A higher initial angle of orientation and more dorsoventral bulging produces a faster muscle contraction but results in a lower amount of force production. It is hypothesized that animals employ a variable gearing mechanism that allows self-regulation of force and velocity to meet the mechanical demands of the contraction. When a pennate muscle is subjected to a low force, resistance to width changes in the muscle cause it to rotate which consequently produce a higher architectural gear ratio (AGR) (high velocity). However, when subject to a high force, the perpendicular fiber force component overcomes the resistance to width changes and the muscle compresses producing a lower AGR (capable of maintaining a higher force output).

Most fishes bend as a simple, homogenous beam during swimming via contractions of longitudinal red muscle fibers and obliquely oriented white muscle fibers within the segmented axial musculature. The fiber strain (εf) experienced by the longitudinal red muscle fibers is equivalent to the longitudinal strain (εx). The deeper white muscle fibers fishes show diversity in arrangement. These fibers are organized into cone-shaped structures and attach to connective tissue sheets known as myosepta; each fiber shows a characteristic dorsoventral (α) and mediolateral (φ) trajectory. The segmented architecture theory predicts that, εx > εf. This phenomenon results in an architectural gear ratio, determined as longitudinal strain divided by fiber strain (εx / εf), greater than one and longitudinal velocity amplification; furthermore, this emergent velocity amplification may be augmented by variable architectural gearing via mesolateral and dorsoventral shape changes, a pattern seen in pennate muscle contractions. A red-to-white gearing ratio (red εf / white εf) captures the combined effect of the longitudinal red muscle fiber and oblique white muscle fiber strains.

Simple bending behavior in homogenous beams suggests ε increases with distance from the neutral axis (z). This poses a problem to animals, such as fishes and salamanders, which undergo undulatory movement. Muscle fibers are constrained by the length-tension and force-velocity curves. Furthermore, it has been hypothesized that muscle fibers recruited for a particular task must operate within an optimal range of strains (ε) and contractile velocities to generate peak force and power respectively. Non-uniform ε generation during undulatory movement would force differing muscle fibers recruited for the same task to operate on differing portions of the length-tension and force-velocity curves; performance would not be optimal. Alexander predicted that the dorsoventral (α) and mediolateral (φ) orientation of the white fibers of the fish axial musculature may allow more uniform strain across varying mesolateral fiber distances. Unfortunately, the white muscle fiber musculature of fishes is too complex to study uniform strain generation; however, Azizi *et al.* studied this phenomenon using a simplified salamander model.

Siren lacertian, an aquatic salamander, utilizes swimming motions similar to the aforementioned fishes yet contains hypaxial muscle fibers (which generate bending) characterized by a simpler organization. The hypaxial muscle fibers of S. lacertian are obliquely oriented, but have a near zero mediolateral (φ) trajectory and a constant doroslateral (α) trajectory within each segment. Therefore, the effect of doroslateral (α) trajectory and the distance between a given hypaxial muscle layer and the neutral axis of bending (z) on muscle fiber strain (ε) can be studied.

Azizi *et al.* found that longitudinal contractions of the constant volume hypaxial muscles were compensated by an increase in the dorsoventral dimensions. Bulging was accompanied by fiber rotation as well as an increase in both α hypaxial fiber trajectory and architectural gear ratio (AGR), a phenomenon also seen in pennate muscle contractions. Azizi *et al.* constructed a mathematical model to predict the final hypaxial fiber angle, AGR and dorsoventral height, where: λx = longitudinal extension ratio of the segment (portortion of final longitudinal length after contraction to initial longitudinal length), β = final fiber angle, γ = initial fiber angle, f = initial fiber length, and εx and εf = longitudinal and fiber strain respectively.

- $\lambda x = \varepsilon x + 1$
- $\lambda f = \varepsilon f + 1$
- $\varepsilon x = \Delta L / Linital$
- Architectural gear ratio = $\varepsilon x / \varepsilon f = [\lambda f(\cos \beta / \cos \gamma) - 1)] / (\lambda f - 1)$
- $\beta = \sin\text{-}1\,(y2 / \lambda ff)$

This relationship shows that AGR increase with an increase in fiber angle from γ to β. In addition, final fiber angle (β) increases with dorsolateral bulging (y) and fiber contraction, but decreases as a function of initial fiber length.

The application of the latter conclusions can be seen in S. lacertian. This organism undulates as a homogenous beam (just as in fishes) during swimming; thus the distance of a muscle fiber from the neutral axis (z) during bending must be greater for external oblique muscle layers (EO) than internal oblique muscle layers (IO). The relationship between the strains (ε) experienced by the EO and IO and their respective z values is given by the following equation: where εEO and εIO = strain of the external and internal oblique muscle layers, and zEO and zIO = distance of the external and internal oblique muscle layers respectively from the neutral axis.

$$\varepsilon EO = \varepsilon IO\ (zEO / zIO)$$

Via this equation, we see that z is directly proportional to ε; the strain experienced by the EO exceeds that of the IO. Azizi *et al.* discovered that the initial hypaxial fiber α trajectory in the EO is greater than that of the IO. Because initial α trajectory is proportional to the AGR, the EO contracts with a greater AGR than the IO. The resulting velocity amplification allows both layers of muscles to operate at similar strains and shortening velocities; this enables the EO and IO to function on comparable portions of the length-tension and force-velocity curves. Muscles recruited for a similar task ought to operate at similar strains and velocities to maximize force and power output. Therefore, variability in AGR within the hypaxial musculature of the Siren lacertian counteracts varying mesolateral fiber distances and optimizes performance. Azizi *et al.* termed this phenomenon as fiber strain homogeneity in segmented musculature.

Muscle Activity

In addition to a rostral to caudal kinematic wave that travels down the animals body during undulatory locomotion, there is also a corresponding wave of muscle activation that travels in the rostro-caudal direction. However, while this pattern is characteristic of undulatory locomotion, it too can vary with environment.

American Eel

Aquatic Locomotion: Electromyogram (EMG) recordings of the American eel reveal a similar pattern of muscle activation during aquatic movement as that of fish. At slow speeds only the most posterior end of the eel's muscles are activated with more anterior muscle recruited at higher speeds. As in many other animals, the muscles activate late in the lengthening phase of the muscle strain cycle, just prior to muscle shortening which is a pattern believed to maximize work output from the muscle.

Terrestrial Locomotion: EMG recordings show a longer absolute duration and duty cycle of muscle activity during locomotion on land. Also, the absolute intensity is much higher while on land which is expected from the increase in gravitational forces acting on the animal. However, the intensity level decreases more posteriorly along the length of the eel's body. Also, the timing of muscle activation shifts to later in the strain cycle of muscle shortening.

Energetics

Animals with elongated bodies and reduced or no legs have evolved differently from their limbed relatives. In the past, some have speculated that this evolution was due to a lower energetic cost associated with limbless locomotion. The biomechanical arguments used to support this rationale include that (1) there is no cost associatied with the vertical displacement of the center of mass typically found with limbed animals, (2) there is no cost associated with accelerating or decelerating limbs, and (3) there is a lower cost for supporting the body. This hypothesis has been studied further by examining the oxygen consumption rates in the snake during different modes of locomotion: lateral undulation, concertina, and sidewinding. The *net cost of transport* (NCT), which indicates the amount of energy required to move a unit of mass a given distance, for a snake moving with a lateral undulatory gait is identical to that of a limbed lizard with the same mass. However, a snake utilizing concertina locomotion produces a much higher net cost of transport, while sidewinding actually produces a lower net cost of transport. Therefore, the different modes of locomotion are of primary importance when determining energetic cost. The reason that lateral undulation has the same energetic efficiency as limbed animals and not less, as hypothesized earlier, might be due to the additional biomechanical cost associated with this type of movement due to the force needed to bend the body laterally, push its sides against a vertical surface, and overcome sliding friction.

Neuromuscular System

Intersegmental Coordination

Wavelike motor pattern typically arise from a series of coupled segmental oscillator. Each segmental oscillator is capable of producing a rhythmic motor output in the absence of sensory feedback. One such example is the half center oscillator which consist of two neurons that are mutually inhibitory and produce activity 180 degrees out of phase. The phase relationships between these oscillators are established by the emergent properties of the oscillators and the coupling between them. Forward swimming can by accomplished by a series of coupled oscillators in which the anterior oscillators have a shorter endogenous frequency than the posterior oscillators. In this case, all oscillators will be driven at the same period but the anterior oscillators will lead in phase. In addition, the phase relations can be established by asymmetries in the couplings between oscillators or by sensory feedback mechanisms.

- Leech: The leech moves by producing dorsoventral undulations. The phase lags between body segments is about 20 degrees and independent of cycle period. Thus, both hemisegments of the oscillator fire synchronously to produce a contraction. Only the ganglia rostral to the midpoint are capable of producing oscillation individually. There is U-shaped gradient in endogenous segment oscillation as well with the highest oscillations frequencies occurring near the middle of the animal. Although the couplings between neurons spans six segments in both the anterior and posterior direction, there are asymmetries between the various interconnections because the oscillators are active at three different phases. Those that are active in the 0 degree phase project only in the descending direction while those projecting in the ascending direction are active at 120 degrees or 240 degrees. In addition, sensory feedback from the environment may contribute to resultant phase lag.

- Lamprey: The lamprey moves using lateral undulation and consequently left and right motor hemisegments are active 180 degrees out of phase. Also, it has been found that the endogenous frequency of the more anterior oscillators is higher than that of the more posterior ganglia. In addition, inhibitory interneurons in the lamprey project 14-20 segments caudally but have short rostral projections. Sensory feedback may be important for appropriately responding to perturbations, but seems to be less important for maintaince of appropriate phase relations.

Robotics

Based on biologically hypothesized connections of the central pattern generator in the salamander, a robotic system has been created which exhibits the same characteristics of the actual animal. Electrophysiology studies have shown that stimulation of the mesencephalic locomotor region (MLR) located in the brain of the salamander produce different gaits, swimming or walking, depending on intensity level. Similarly, the CPG model in the robot can exhibit walking at low levels of tonic drive and swimming at high levels of tonic drive. The model is based on the four assumptions that:

- Tonic stimulation of the body CPG produces spontaneous traveling waves. When the limb CPG is activated it overrides the body CPG.
- The strength of the coupling from the limb to the body CPG is stronger than that from body to limb.
- Limb oscillators saturate and stop oscillating at higher tonic drives.
- Limb oscillators have lower intrinsic frequencies than body CPGs at the same tonic drive.

This model encompasses the basic features of salamander locomotion.

References

- Cavagna, G. A.; Saibene, F. P.; Margaria, R. (1964). "Mechanical Work in Running". Journal of applied physiology. 19: 249–256. PMID 14155290
- Samra HA, Specker B (July 2007). "Walking Age Does Not Explain Term vs. Preterm Differences in Bone Geometry". J Pediatr. 151 (1): 61–6, 66.e1–2. PMC 2031218. PMID 17586192. doi:10.1016/j.jpeds.2007.02.033
- "Spanner crab Ranina ranina". Fishing and Aquaculture. New South Wales Department of Primary Industries. 2005. Retrieved January 4, 2009
- Tolley, Rodney (2003). Sustainable transport: planning for walking and cycling in urban environments. Woodhead Publishing. p. 72. ISBN 1-85573-614-4
- Church TS, Earnest CP, Morss GM (2013-03-25). "Field testing of physiological responses associated with Nordic Walking". Res Q Exerc Sport. 73: 296–300. PMID 12230336. doi:10.1080/02701367.2002.10609023
- Nicola, T. L.; Jewison, D. J. (2012). "The Anatomy and Biomechanics of Running". Clinical Journal of Sports Medicine. 31: 187–201. doi:10.1016/j.csm.2011.10.001
- Alpha, Rob (2015). What Is Sport: A Controversial Essay About Why Humans Play Sports. BookBaby. ISBN 9781483555232
- "Relationship of walking to mortality among U.S. adults". Centers for Disease Control. 20 May 2011. Archived from the original on 29 January 2013. Retrieved 16 October 2013
- Davis, G.J. (1980). "Mechanisms of Selected Knee Injuries". Journal of the American Physical Therapy Association. 60: 1590–95
- Lindsay, Everett H.; Fahlbusch, Volker; Mein, Pierre (2013), European Neogene Mammal Chronology, Nato Science Series A, 180, Springer Science & Business Media, p. 658, ISBN 9781489925138
- Anderson, T (1996). "Biomechanics and Running Economy". Sports Medicine. 22 (2): 76–89. doi:10.2165/00007256-199622020-00003
- Nielsen, R.O (2013). "Classifying running-related injuries based upon etiology, with emphasis on volume and pace". International Journal of Sports Physical Therapy. 8 (2): 172–9

- King, R.S. (2013). "BiLBIQ: A Biologically Inspired Robot with Walking and Rolling Locomotion". Biosystems and Biorobotics. 2. Springer, Verlag, Berlin, Heidelberg. ISBN 978-3-642-34681-1. doi:10.1007/978-3-642-34682-8
- "Merriam's Kangaroo Rat Dipodomys merriami". U. S. Bureau of Land Management web site. Bureau of Land Management. Retrieved 2014-03-26
- Gao, X.; Jiang, L. (2004). "Biophysics: water-repellent legs of water striders". Nature. 432 (7013): 36–36. doi:10.1038/432036a
- Brady, Richard M. (1993). "Torque and switching in the bacterial flagellar motor. An electrostatic model.". Biophysical Journal. 64: 961–973. Bibcode:1993BpJ....64..961B. doi:10.1016/S0006-3495(93)81462-0
- Harkness, John E.; Wagner, Joseph E. (1995). The Biology and Medicine of Rabbits and Rodents. Williams & Wilkins. pp. 30–39. ISBN 0-683-03919-9
- Stewart, D. (2006-08-01). "A Bird Like No Other". National Wildlife. National Wildlife Federation. Archived from the original on 2012-02-09. Retrieved 2014-05-30

4

A Comprehensive Study of Sports Biomechanics

Sports biomechanics is the analysis of any form of physical movement displayed in sports in general. Kinematics and kinetics are two important aspects of sports biomechanics. The aspects elucidated in this chapter are of vital importance, and provide a better understanding of biomechanics.

Sports Biomechanics

Sports biomechanics is a quantitative based study and analysis of professional athletes and sports' activities in general. It can simply be described as the Physics of Sports. In this subfield of biomechanics the laws of mechanics are applied in order to gain a greater understanding of athletic performance through mathematical modeling, computer simulation and measurement. Biomechanics is the study of the structure and function of biological systems by means of the methods of "mechanics." – which is the branch of physics involving analysis of the actions of forces. Within "mechanics" there are two sub-fields of study: statics, which is the study of systems that are in a state of constant motion either at rest (with no motion) or moving with a constant velocity; and dynamics, which is the study of systems in motion in which acceleration is present, which may involve kinematics (the study of the motion of bodies with respect to time, displacement, velocity, and speed of movement either in a straight line or in a rotary direction) and kinetics (the study of the forces associated with motion, including forces causing motion and forces resulting from motion).

Theoretical Sports Biomechanics

- Computer simulation
- Engineering mechanics
- Muscle mechanics
- Motor coordination
- Kinematics
- Inverse dynamics

- Statics
- Kinetics
- Velocity
- Displacement
- Acceleration
- Moment of Inertia
- Torque
- Digital filters

Experimental Sports Biomechanics

Methods:

- 3D Motion capture analysis
- Force plates
- Force transducers
- Strain gauges
- Anthropometric measurements (mathematical models)
- Surface EMG (Electromyography)

Research and Applications

- Golf swing
- Tennis
- Gymnastics
- Track and field
- Running blades
- Swimming
- Diving
- Skiing
- Trampoline
- Rowing
- Baseball

- Figure Skating
- Exergaming design and evaluation
- Movement Assessment
- Olympic weightlifting
- Powerlifting

Golf Stroke Mechanics

Golf stroke mechanics is the means by which golfers make decisions (selecting clubs, selecting shots) and execute them (making shots) in the sport of golf. For all golfers, it consists of a pre-stroke, in which golfers choose which club they want and their stance, and the actual stroke. The stroke is a complex motion and there is still disagreement on what constitutes a "good" golf swing. In *Work and Power Analysis of the Golf Swing*, Nesbit and Serrano suggest the golf swing has been studied by scientists and mathematicians who have developed various equations to help explain the complexity of the swing. It is generally agreed that a successful and consistent golf swing requires precise timing and mechanics, from the grip and position of one's fingers, to the position and movement of the feet. At any moment of the swing, whether back-swing, downswing, or upswing, something can go wrong that will throw off the whole body and result in a mishit. The entire swing motion should move on a plane in a fluid manner. The plane can be characterized as horizontal or vertical.

Complex Motion

The goal of the golf swing is to direct as much kinetic energy as possible into the club head so when it comes into contact with the ball, all of the energy will transfer to the ball, sending it into flight. The complex motion of the body first starts with the stance. This is critical to make sure the golfer has a low center of gravity to remain balanced throughout the swing path. The swing starts with the arms moving back in a straight line. When the club head reaches the level of the hip, two things happen: there is a stern wrist cock that acts as a hinge along with the left knee (for a right handed swing), building up its torque by moving into the same line as the belly button before the start of the upswing. As the swing continues to the top of the backswing (again for right-handed golf swing), the golfer's left arm should be perfectly straight and his right arm should be hinged at the elbow. The downswing begins with the hips and the lower body rather than the arms and upper body, with emphasis on the wrist cock. As the golfer's hips turn into the shot, the right elbow will drop straight down, hugging the right side of the golfer's torso. As the right elbow drops, the wrists begin to snap through from the wrist cock in the backswing. A solid extension of the arms and good transfer of body should put the golfer leaning up on his right toe, balanced, with the golf club resting on the back of the golfers neck. Importantly, all of the movements occur with precise timing, while the head remains completely still with eyes focused on the ball throughout the entire swing.

Musculature

A golf stroke uses muscles on core (especially erector spinae muscles and latissimus dorsi muscle when turning), hamstring, shoulder and wrist. Stronger muscles on wrist can prevent wrists from being twisted at swings, while stronger shoulders increase the turning force. Weak wrists can also deliver the impacts to elbows and even neck and lead to injury of them. (When a muscle contracts, it pulls equally from both ends and, in order to have movement at only one end of the muscle, other muscles must come into play to stabilize the bone to which the other end of the muscle is attached.) Golf is a unilateral exercise that can break body balances, requiring exercises to keep the balance in muscles. A recommended exercise is free weight, an exercise not reliant on machines to stimulate and balance the fine muscles.

Pre-swing

Posture

- A good golf swing starts with proper posture. Having a proper posture means standing upright with a relatively straight back and slightly bent knees. When a golfer takes the stance, the width of the stance should be about shoulder wide and arms should be hanging free.
- Slightly more weight is placed on the front foot for short irons, with balance shifting onto both feet through the middle irons until weight is distributed fairly evenly for long irons and woods.

Alignment

- At address the body is positioned parallel to the target line, although stance can be adjusted for different shots; in general the body and stance should be parallel to the target line.
- The ball is positioned near the center of the player's stance for short irons, moving forward of center through the middle and long irons until it is opposite the heel of the front foot for woods.

Grip

- There are several choices with regard to gripping the club. Generally one of the following three will be used:

- Vardon overlap (or overlapping) grip: Named for Harry Vardon, the man who popularized it, the little finger of the trailing hand (the non-dominant hand) is placed between the index and middle finger of the lead hand (the dominant hand). The lead-hand thumb fits along the lifeline of the trailing hand.
- Interlocking grip: The little finger of the trailing hand is intertwined with the index finger of the lead hand. The lead-hand thumb fits in the lifeline of the trailing hand.
- Ten finger (or baseball) grip: The little finger of the trailing hand is placed close to the index finger of the lead hand. The lead-hand thumb is covered with the lifeline of the trailing hand.

Timing

Timing is the most critical element of the golf swing because it connects all of the different moving parts of the body into one motion. "On the backswing aka the first part of the swing, the order of movement goes like this: hands, arms, shoulders, hips" (*Ben Hogan: Five Lessons: the Modern Fundamentals*). The downswing (the second part of the swing) is initiated by the unwinding of the hips. Then the shoulders and arms follow.

Power

The golf swing is capable of producing great force, though it takes practice to be able to effectively utilize it in a productive manner. Most amateur golfers try to get as much power as possible, and try to hit the ball as far as possible but this is not an appropriate approach for an amateur. The power of the golf swing is not unlocked by muscle or by fastest club head speed, but by the precise timing and mechanics of a motion that has to be put together in harmony. With more power, comes the necessity for more control over the body that a golfer must have to control the motions of the swing. "Strength and inertial variations seem more likely than size to account for long and short hitting".

Stroke Types

Chip

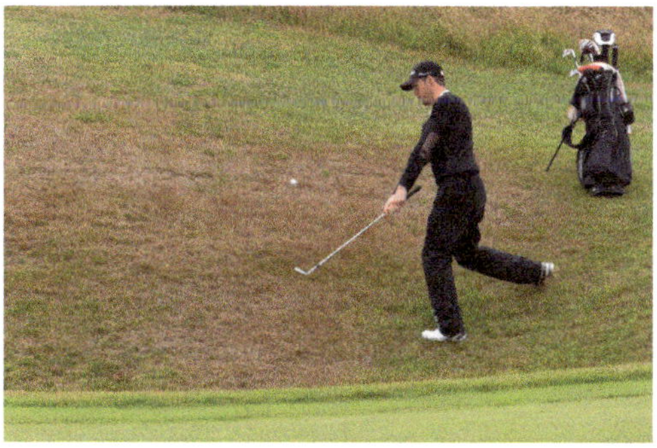

Callum Aird's chipping 2013

The chip is a type of shot generally used from short range around the green usually under 40 yards. Although any club may be used, and there are specialist chipping clubs (or chippers) available, a short iron or wedge is most common. The goal of the chip is to land the ball safely on the green and let it roll out towards the hole.

Pitch

A "pitch shot" is a shot played with a high lofted club, typically a pitching wedge, utility wedge or sand wedge, with lofts ranging from 56° to 62° degrees. These high lofted clubs are designed to hit the ball high from short distances, usually from 40-50 yards (30-50 meters) and closer.

Putt

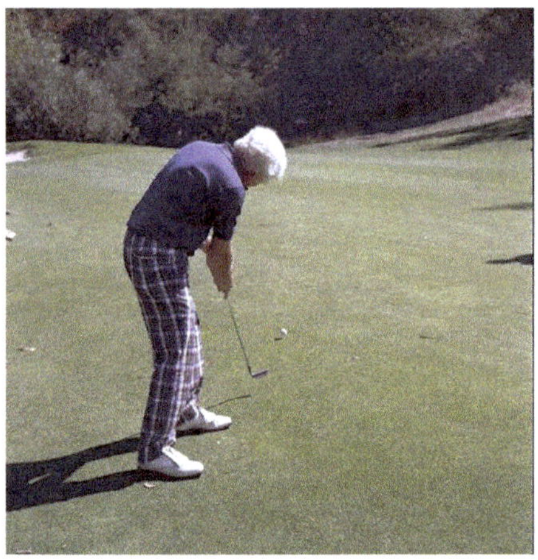

The putt by a right-handed golfer.

The putt is used for putting the ball in the hole or closer to the hole (as in lagging) from the green or the fringe of the green. The putter is used for the putt. The golfer adjusts his/her putt to fit the circumstances of the play such as distance to the hole and slope of the green. The face of the club starts square to the target line. The club goes straight back and straight through along the same path like a pendulum. One strategy is to aim the ball 10% past the hole. Another is to look at the hole for long putts instead of the ball.

Shots

List of Shots

- A *drive* is a long-distance shot played from the tee box, intended to move the ball a great distance down the fairway towards the green.
- An *approach* shot is made with the intention of placing the ball on the green. The term "approach" typically refers to a second or subsequent shot with a shorter-range iron depending on the distance required.

- A *lay-up* shot is made from the fairway after the drive, but intended to travel a shorter distance than might normally be expected and/or with a higher degree of accuracy, due to intervening circumstances. Most often, a lay-up shot is made to avoid hitting the ball into a hazard placed in the fairway, or to position the ball in a more favorable position on the fairway for the next shot.
- A *chip* is a very short shot played from near the green, generally made with an abbreviated swing motion. Chip shots are used as short approach shots to the green.
- A *pitch* is slightly longer than a chip shot and thus requires a slightly larger swing. It is generally hit with a lofted club and expected to stop fairly quickly once reaching the green.
- A *bunker shot* is a shot played from a sand trap. It is hit with a lofted wedge and is intended to hit the ball high so that it can carry over the lip of the bunker while still staying on the green.
- A *flop* shot is when a player opens the club face on a chip shot to get the ball to fly over an obstacle and stop quickly or spin back once it hits the ground.
- A *putt* is a shot designed to roll the ball along the ground. It is normally made on the putting green using a putter, though other clubs may be used to achieve the same effect in different situations. A *lag* is a long putt designed less to try to place the ball in the cup than to simply move the ball closer to the hole for an easier putt into the hole.

Secondary Characteristics

- A *draw* is a stroke played with the effect that, for a right-handed player, the ball moves from right to left during flight. Conversely the ball will move from left to right for a left-handed player. These characteristics are achieved with sidespin by either an in-to-out swingpath or a closed clubface, relative to the swingpath, at impact.
- A *fade* is a stroke played with the effect that, for a right-handed player, the ball moves from left to right during flight. Conversely the ball will move from right to left for a left-handed player. These characteristics are achieved by having either an out-to-in swingpath or an open clubface, relative to the swingpath, at impact, again due to sidespin.
- A *punch* or *knock-down* shot is one with a low trajectory, that is employed when hitting into the wind or in order to avoid hitting the ball into overhead obstructions. This stroke is achieved by keeping the weight forward and the hands ahead of the clubhead through impact.

Misplayed Shots

- A *hook* occurs when the clubface is closed relative to the swingpath or with an inside-out swingpath and thus flies severely from right to left for a right-handed player, or vice versa for a left-handed player. Skilled players can hook the ball at will, but most commonly it is a misplayed shot that often has negative consequences.
- A *slice* occurs when the clubface is open relative to the swingpath or with an outside-in swingpath and thus flies severely from left to right for a right-handed player, or vice versa for a left-handed player. Skilled players can slice the ball at will, but most commonly it is a misplayed shot that often has negative consequences.
- A *push* is a ball whose flight path is straight, with negligible sidespin, that ends up right of the target. The incidence angle of the clubface is x° to the right of the target, and where the path of the clubface is also x° to the right of the target (inside to outside path).
- A *pull* is a ball whose flight path is straight, with negligible sidespin that ends up left of the target. The incidence angle of the clubface is x° to the left of the target, and where the path of the clubface is also x° to the left of the target (outside to inside path).
- A *shank* occurs when the ball is struck on the hosel of the club, and thus flies at a sharp angle to the right of the intended direction (or vice versa for a left-handed player).
- A *thin* shot occurs when the forward edge of the clubhead strikes the ball too high, causing the shot to fly low, sometimes even causing it to travel across the ground, and usually comes up short of the target.
- A *phin* is an off target shot similar to a thin but it fishtails on landing.
- A *top* occurs when the player strikes the top half of the golf ball causing it to dribble along the ground and come up severely short of the intended target.
- A *fat* shot occurs when the forward edge of the clubhead strikes the ground behind the ball first, causing the shot to come up short of the target.
- A *pop-up (or sky)* occurs when the ball strikes too highly on the clubface, causing the shot to travel very high, leaving it well short of its intended target.
- A *whiff (or air shot)* occurs when the golfer swings and misses the ball.
- A *duff* occurs when the golfer makes contact with the top half of the ball on follow through and then it proceeds to bounce along the ground or when the golfer *chunks* the golf ball causing it to bounce

Other Definitions

- *Backspin* is imparted due to the golf club's loft and the clubhead speed at impact.
- *Sidespin* is imparted due to the non-perpendicularity of the golf club or the path of the clubhead.

Front Crawl

The front crawl or forward crawl, also known as the Australian crawl or American crawl, is a swimming stroke usually regarded as the fastest of the four front primary strokes. As such, the front crawl stroke is almost universally used during a freestyle swimming competition, and hence freestyle is used metonymically for the front crawl. It is one of two long axis strokes, the other one being the backstroke. Unlike the backstroke, the butterfly stroke, and the breaststroke, the front crawl is not regulated by the FINA. This style is sometimes referred to as the Australian crawl although this can sometimes refer to a more specific variant of front crawl.

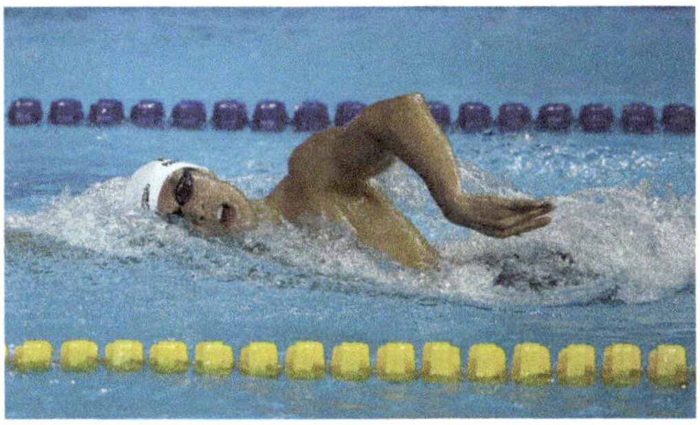

Swimmer breathing during front crawl

Ergonomics

The face-down swimming position allows for a good range of motion of the arm in the water, as compared to the *backstroke*, where the hands cannot be moved easily along the back of the spine. The above-water recovery of the stroke reduces drag, compared to the underwater recovery of *breaststroke*. The alternating arms also allow some rolling movement of the body for an easier recovery compared to, for example, *butterfly*. Finally, the alternating arm stroke makes for a relatively constant speed throughout the cycle.

History

The "front crawl" style has been in use since ancient times. There is an Egyptian bas relief piece dating to 2000 BCE showing it in use.

In the Western world, the stroke, which would later be refined into the modern front crawl, was first seen in a swimming race held in 1844 in London, where it was swum by Northern Native Americans. The Anishinaabe Flying Gull and Tobacco had been invited by the British Swimming Society to give an exhibition at the swimming baths in High Holborn. They raced against each other for a silver medal to be presented by the society, which was won by Flying Gull. English gentlemen, however, considered this style, with its considerable splashing and "grotesque antics", to be barbarically "un-European" and the British continued to swim only the breaststroke in competition.

Sometime around 1873, British swimmer John Arthur Trudgen learned the front crawl from native South Americans during a trip to Argentina. However, Trudgen applied the more common sidestroke (scissor) kick instead of the flutter kick used by the Native Americans. This hybrid stroke was called the Trudgen stroke. Because of its speed, this stroke quickly became popular.

This style was further improved by the Australian champion swimmer, Richmond "Dick" Cavill (the son of swimming instructor Professor Richard "Frederick" Cavill) who developed the stroke with his brother "Tums". They were later inspired by Alick Wickham, a young Solomon Islander living in Sydney who swam a version of the crawl stroke that was popular in his home island at Roviana lagoon. The Cavills then modified their swimming stroke using this as inspiration and this modified Trudgen stroke became known as the "Australian crawl".

The American swimmer Charles Daniels then made modifications to a six-beat kick, thereby creating the "American crawl".

Technique

The starting position for front crawl is known as the "streamline" position. The swimmer starts on the stomach with both arms stretched out to the front and both legs extended to the back.

Arm Movement

The arm movements of the front crawl provide most of the forward motion. The arms alternate from side to side, so while one arm is pulling and pushing under the water, the other arm is recovering above the water. The move can be separated into four parts: the downsweep, the insweep, the upsweep, and the recovery. Each complete arm movement is referred to as a stroke; one stroke with each arm forms a stroke cycle.

From the initial position, the arm sinks slightly lower and the palm of the hand turns 45 degrees with the thumb side of the palm towards the bottom, to catch the water and prepare for the pull. The pull movement follows a semicircle, with the elbow higher than the hand, and the hand pointing towards the body center and downward. The semicircle ends in front of the chest at the beginning of the ribcage.

The push pushes the palm backward through the water underneath the body at the beginning and at the side of the body at the end of the push.

This pull and push is also known as the S-curve.

Some time after the beginning of the pull, the other arm begins its recovery. The recovery moves the elbow in a semicircle in a vertical plane in the swimming direction. The lower arm and the hand are completely relaxed and *hang* down from the elbow close to the water surface and close to the swimmer's body. The beginning of the recovery looks similar to pulling the hand out of the back pocket of a pair of pants, with the small finger upwards. Further into the recovery phase, the hand movement has been compared to pulling up a center zip on a wetsuit. The recovering hand moves forward, with the fingers trailing downward, just above the surface of the water. In the middle of the recovery one shoulder is rotated forward into the air while the other is pointing backwards to avoid drag due to the large frontal area which at this specific time is not covered by the arm. To rotate the shoulder, some twist their torso while others also rotate everything down to their feet.

Beginners often make the mistake of not relaxing the arm during the recovery and of moving the hand too high and too far away from the body, in some cases even higher than the elbow. In these cases, drag and incidental muscle effort is increased at the expense of speed. Beginners often forget to use their shoulders to let the hand enter as far forward as possible. Some say the hand should enter the water thumb first, reducing drag through possible turbulence, others say the middle finger is first with the hand precisely bent down, giving thrust right from the start. At the beginning of the pull, the hand acts like a wing and is moved slower than the swimmer while at the end it acts like an oar and is moved faster than the swimmer.

Leg Movement

There are several kicks that can be used with the upper body action of the front crawl. Because the front crawl is most commonly used in freestyle competitions, all of these kicks are legal.

The most usual leg movement with the front crawl is called the flutter kick. The legs move alternately, with one leg kicking downward while the other leg moves upward. While the legs provide only a small part of the overall speed, they are important to stabilize the body position. This lack of balance is apparent when using a pull buoy to neutralize the leg action.

The leg in the initial position bends very slightly at the knees, and then kicks the lower leg and the foot downwards similar to kicking a football. The legs may be bent inward (or occasionally outward) slightly. After the kick, the straight leg moves back up. A frequent mistake of beginners is to bend the legs too much or to kick too much out of the water.

Ideally, there are 6 kicks per cycle (the stroke so performed is called the *American crawl*), although it is also possible to use 8, 4, or even 2 kicks; Franziska van Almsick, for example, swam very successfully with 4 kicks per cycle. When one arm is pushed down, the opposite leg needs to do a downward kick also, to fix the body orientation, because this happens shortly after the body rotation.

Breathing

Normally, the face is in the water during front crawl with eyes looking at the lower part of the wall in front of the pool, with the waterline between the brow line and the hairline. Breaths are taken through the mouth by turning the head to the side of a recovering arm at the beginning of the recovery, and breathing *in the triangle between the upper arm, lower arm, and the waterline*. The swimmer's forward movement will cause a bow wave with a trough in the water surface near the ears. After turning the head, a breath can be taken in this trough without the need to move the mouth above the average water surface. A thin film of water running down the head can be blown away just before the intake. The head is rotated back at the end of the recovery and points down and forward again when the recovered hand enters the water. The swimmer breathes out through mouth and nose until the next breath. Breathing out through the nose may help to prevent water from entering the nose. Swimmers with allergies exacerbated by time in the pool should not expect exhaling through the nose to completely prevent intranasal irritation.

Standard swimming calls for one breath every third arm recovery or every 1.5 cycles, alternating the sides for breathing. Some swimmers instead take a breath every cycle, i.e., every second arm recovery, breathing always to the same side. Most competition swimmers will breathe every other stroke, or once a cycle, to a preferred side. However some swimmers can breathe comfortably to both sides. Sprinters will often breathe a predetermined number of times in an entire race. Elite sprinters will breathe once or even no times during a fifty-metre race. For a one hundred metre race sprinters will often breathe every four strokes, once every two cycles, or will start with every four strokes and finish with every two strokes. In water polo and water rescue, the head is often kept out of the water completely for better visibility and easier breathing, at the price of a much steeper body position and higher drag.

Body Movement

The body rotates about its long axis with every arm stroke so that the shoulder of the recovering arm is higher than the shoulder of the pushing/pulling arm. This makes the recovery much easier and reduces the need to turn the head to breathe. As one shoulder is out of the water, it reduces drag, and as it falls it aids the arm catching the water; as the other shoulder rises it aids the arm at end of the push to leave the water.

Side-to-side movement is kept to a minimum: one of the main functions of the leg kick is to maintain the line of the body.

Racing: turn and finish

The front crawl swimmer uses a tumble turn (also known as a *flip turn*) to reverse directions in minimal time. The swimmer swims close to the wall as quickly as possible. In the swimming position with one arm forward and one arm to the back, the swimmer does not recover one arm, but rather uses the pull/push of the other arm to initialize a somersault with the knees straight to the body. At the end of the somersault the feet are at the wall, and the swimmer is on his or her back with the hands over the head. The swimmer then pushes off the wall while turning sideways to lie on the breast. After a brief gliding phase, the swimmer starts with either a flutter kick or a butterfly kick before surfacing no more than 15 m from the wall.

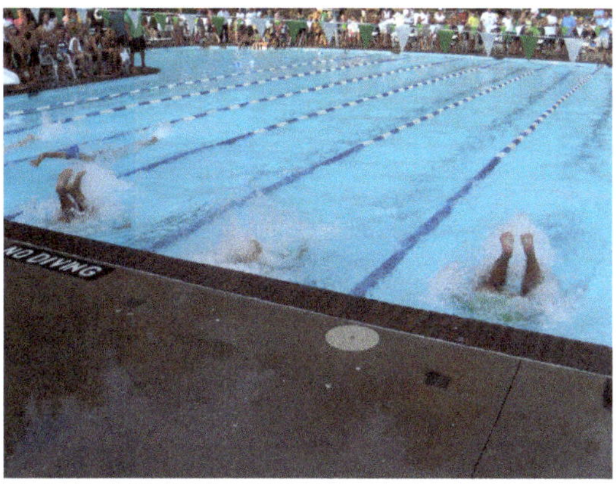

Swimmers turning during a front crawl race

A variant of the tumble turn is to make a somersault earlier with straight legs, throwing the legs toward the wall and gliding to the wall. This has a small risk of injury because the legs could hit another swimmer or the wall.

For the finish the swimmer has to touch the wall with any body part, usually the hand. Most swimmers sprint the finish as quickly as possible, which usually includes reducing their breathing rate.

Training Drills

A variation of front crawl often used in training involves only one arm moving at any one time, while the other arm rests and is stretched out at the front. This style is called a "catch up" stroke because the moving hand touches, or "catches up" to the stationary one before the stationary hand begins its motion. Catch up requires more strength for swimming because the hand is beginning the pull from a stationary position rather than a dynamic one. This style is slower than the regular front crawl and is rarely used competitively; however, it is often used for training purposes by swimmers, as it increases the body's awareness of being streamlined in the water. Total Immersion is a similar technique.

The side swimming, or six kicks per stroke, variation is used in training to improve swimmers' balance and rotation and help them learn to breathe on both sides. Swimmers stretch one arm out in front of their bodies, and one on their sides. They then kick for six counts and then take a stroke to switch sides and continue alternating with six kicks in between.

Another training variation involves swimming with clenched fists, which forces swimmers to use more forearm strength to propel them forward.

References

- Hill, Pete (2008). The Complete Guide to Climbing and Mountaineering. Cincinnati, OH 45236: David&Charles. p. 94. ISBN 978-0-7153-2842-2
- "Bouldering: Understanding and Managing Climbing on Small Rock Formations" (PDF). The Access Fund. 2006. Retrieved 4 August 2013
- Torres-Oviedo, G.; Ting, LH. (Oct 2007). "Muscle synergies characterizing human postural responses". J Neurophysiol. 98 (4): 2144–56. PMID 17652413. doi:10.1152/jn.01360.2006
- Gadd, Will; Roger Chayer (November 2003). Ice & Mixed Climbing: Modern Technique (First ed.). Mountaineers Books. ISBN 0-89886-769-X
- "Lucid Dreaming, new extreme boulder problem at the Buttermilks, Bishop". PlanetMountain. 31 March 2010. Retrieved 11 August 2013
- Nesbit & Serrano, Steven M. & Monika. "Work and Power Analysis of the Golf Swing" (PDF). Journal of Sports Science and Medicine. Retrieved October 10, 2005
- Steven M. Cox and Kris Fulsaas, ed. (2003) [1960]. Mountaineering: The Freedom of the Hills (7th ed.). Seattle: The Mountaineers Books. ISBN 978-0898868289
- Dentico, Michael J. (10 Aug 2016). "Trump Tower Climber Stephen Rogata Captured By NYPD After Reaching 21st Floor". Inquisitr. Retrieved 10 Aug 2016
- Liesker, H.; Brenner, E.; Smeets, JB. (Aug 2009). "Combining eye and hand in search is suboptimal". Exp Brain Res. 197 (4): 395–401. PMC 2721960. PMID 19590859. doi:10.1007/s00221-009-1928-9
- Beal, Peter (2011). Bouldering: Movement, Tactics, and Problem Solving. The Mountaineers Books. ISBN 9781594855016
- "From"Weissmuller to Spitz;"The History and Background of the Olympic Game". International Swimming Hall of Fame. Retrieved 23 January 2014

Permissions

All chapters in this book are published with permission under the Creative Commons Attribution Share Alike License or equivalent. Every chapter published in this book has been scrutinized by our experts. Their significance has been extensively debated. The topics covered herein carry significant information for a comprehensive understanding. They may even be implemented as practical applications or may be referred to as a beginning point for further studies.

We would like to thank the editorial team for lending their expertise to make the book truly unique. They have played a crucial role in the development of this book. Without their invaluable contributions this book wouldn't have been possible. They have made vital efforts to compile up to date information on the varied aspects of this subject to make this book a valuable addition to the collection of many professionals and students.

This book was conceptualized with the vision of imparting up-to-date and integrated information in this field. To ensure the same, a matchless editorial board was set up. Every individual on the board went through rigorous rounds of assessment to prove their worth. After which they invested a large part of their time researching and compiling the most relevant data for our readers.

The editorial board has been involved in producing this book since its inception. They have spent rigorous hours researching and exploring the diverse topics which have resulted in the successful publishing of this book. They have passed on their knowledge of decades through this book. To expedite this challenging task, the publisher supported the team at every step. A small team of assistant editors was also appointed to further simplify the editing procedure and attain best results for the readers.

Apart from the editorial board, the designing team has also invested a significant amount of their time in understanding the subject and creating the most relevant covers. They scrutinized every image to scout for the most suitable representation of the subject and create an appropriate cover for the book.

The publishing team has been an ardent support to the editorial, designing and production team. Their endless efforts to recruit the best for this project, has resulted in the accomplishment of this book. They are a veteran in the field of academics and their pool of knowledge is as vast as their experience in printing. Their expertise and guidance has proved useful at every step. Their uncompromising quality standards have made this book an exceptional effort. Their encouragement from time to time has been an inspiration for everyone.

The publisher and the editorial board hope that this book will prove to be a valuable piece of knowledge for students, practitioners and scholars across the globe.

Index